M. HENRY WILLIAMS, Jr., M.D.

Professor of Medicine, Albert Einstein College of Medicine
Director, Chest Service, Bronx Municipal Hospital Center
Bronx, New York

Essentials of
PULMONARY
MEDICINE

W. B. SAUNDERS COMPANY

Philadelphia   London   Toronto
Mexico City   Rio de Janeiro   Sydney   Tokyo

W. B. Saunders Company: West Washington Square
Philadelphia, PA 19105

1 St. Anne's Road
Eastbourne, East Sussex BN21 3UN, England

1 Goldthorne Avenue
Toronto, Ontario M8Z 5T9, Canada

Cedro 512
Mexico 4, D.F., Mexico

Rua Coronel Cabrita, 8
Sao Cristovao Caixa Postal 21176
Rio de Janeiro, Brazil

9 Waltham Street
Artarmon, N.S.W. 2064, Australia

Ichibancho, Central Bldg., 22-1
Chiyoda-ku, Tokyo 102, Japan

Library of Congress Cataloging in Publication Data

Williams, M. Henry (Marshall Henry), 1924–

Essentials of pulmonary medicine.

1. Lungs—Diseases.   I. Title. [DNLM: 1. Respiratory tract
diseases. WF 140 W725e]

RC756.W54   616.2'4   81–50836

ISBN 0–7216–9394–6   AACR2

Essentials of Pulmonary Medicine   ISBN   0-7216-9394-6

Last digit is the print number: 9   8   7   6   5   4   3   2

To Stuart

PREFACE

Although pulmonary medicine is an important specialty within internal medicine and the pulmonary physician has extensive knowledge of the lung and of respiratory disease as well as special skills, such as the ability to perform bronchoscopy, most patients with pulmonary disease can and should be treated by general medical internists. These physicians must have a working knowledge of pulmonary function, they should incorporate spirometric tests in the evaluation and treatment of their patients, and they should understand the implications of measurements of arterial blood gases. In this book, major emphasis has been placed on the common pulmonary problems, particularly obstructive airways disease; pulmonary infections, including tuberculosis; and other disorders that can be managed entirely by the general physician. Other diseases and topics have been included either because of their intrinsic interest or because general physicians should recognize them and know when special help and technology should be sought.

The material has been presented both from the standpoint of the problems that the patient presents to the physician and as a more detailed discussion of the common diseases. A short bibliography has been included with each chapter if more detailed information is needed. It is hoped that the book may be read with interest and profit and that it may also serve as a reference. If the effort has been successful, physicians will read the book with sufficient interest to incorporate useful information into their long-term working memory. They will also be able to look up information that is necessary for the management of a specific problem with which they may not be familiar.

I am extremely grateful to the medical students, house officers, and faculty of the Chest Service of the Albert Einstein College of Medicine-Bronx Municipal Hospital Center who have been teaching me Chest Medicine for the past 20 years, especially to Dr. Chang Shim, who read most of the manuscript, and to Dr. Isidore Bobrowitz, who provided the roentgenograms used in Figures 4–3 and 7–1. I am also particularly grateful to Mrs. Angela Palmeri and Dawn Hellwinkel for their expert secretarial support.

Contents

CHAPTER ONE

EVALUATION OF THE PATIENT WITH PULMONARY DISEASE

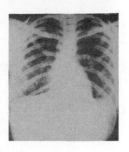

This initial chapter is a description of the important techniques used in evaluating the patient with pulmonary disease: history, physical examination, sputum examination, x-rays, pulmonary function studies, and specialized diagnostic techniques. These techniques will be described in connection with the cause and significance of abnormal findings. This will provide an introduction to the evaluation and exploration of the problems that often cause the patient to seek medical attention and to the approach used by physicians in their own evaluation of patients. More detailed descriptions of disease and a more extensive consideration of some of the major problems encountered in chest medicine will be presented in the coming chapters.

HISTORY

The history represents the focus of the first encounter between patient and physician. Properly obtained, it often provides sufficient information for an accurate diagnosis. In addition, the act of taking a history is the first step in establishing a trusting relationship with the patient. From the history, the physician learns who the patient is and what types of disease he or she is liable to develop.

Cough

Cough is probably the most common symptom present in patients with pulmonary disease and must always be taken seriously. Patients presenting with *acute* development of cough and fever almost always suffer from pulmonary infection. It is particularly important to establish the nature of associated sputum production — the amount and character of the expectorated material. Nonbacterial infections or even bacterial pneumonia can present, at an early stage, with nonproductive cough, but purulent sputum is characteristic of bacterial pneumonia and acute bronchitis. Blood-streaked or rusty sputum is not uncommon in bacterial infection, but expectoration of large amounts of blood is distinctly unusual and suggests the presence of an

1

underlying or more chronic disease, such as bronchiectasis or cavity formation in the lung from tuberculosis or lung abscess. Foul-smelling sputum
signifies anaerobic infection, usually with a lung abscess or bronchiectasis;
and the sudden expectoration of a large amount of sputum suggests the
development of a bronchopleural fistula into an empyema pocket.

In patients with *chronic* symptoms the evaluation of cough becomes
particularly important. In cigarette smokers, a chronic cough is often
considered synonymous with chronic bronchitis; but it is important to
recognize that such patients are also at risk of developing lung cancer, and
any change in the nature or severity of cough requires careful consideration
of additional disease. A smoker who suddenly begins to cough demands the
same diagnostic concern as a nonsmoker. The nature of the sputum is also
important, and hemoptysis must always be considered seriously. Although
patients with chronic bronchitis may occasionally cough up blood, particularly with heavy coughing, the first hemoptysis always requires investigation to exclude more important underlying disease. Generally, if the cause is
not apparent, fiberoptic bronchoscopy must be done. Hemoptysis occurring
in the absence of severe cough is even more significant, suggesting the
presence of either a cavitary lesion in the lung or, if this is not visible on the
x-ray film of the chest, a bronchial adenoma. In the patient with hemoptysis,
it is important to inquire about the source, since many individuals can
describe a sensation, often of warmth, in the area of the tracheobronchial tree
where the blood originates. This may be very helpful in directing further
studies or even in localizing a bleeding tumor. Sometimes bleeding from the
nose or the gastrointestinal tract has to be excluded by careful history and
physical examination.

Paroxysmal dry cough is not an uncommon feature of asthma and may
even outweigh the intensity of dyspnea and wheeze in some patients. Under
these circumstances, careful inquiry into the times during which cough
occurs, associated symptoms, and other characteristic findings of asthma
becomes very important. It should be emphasized that pronounced sputum
eosinophilia, often found in asthma, may be associated with sputum that
appears to be purulent not because of polymorphonuclear leukocytes but
because of the presence of eosinophils. In patients with asthma, cough is
almost always associated with a feeling of chest tightness, and not uncommonly the paroxysms of cough lead to worsening of tightness, wheeze, and
dyspnea.

Patients with pulmonary congestion due to left ventricular failure often
complain of cough in association with dyspnea, particularly at night. The
development of dyspnea and cough an hour or two after lying down is quite
characteristic of pulmonary congestion, whereas patients with chronic obstructive lung disease who develop cough and dyspnea on lying down
generally do so immediately, often with relief after cough and expectoration
of sputum.

Dyspnea

This is the second most important symptom that requires careful evaluation.
Dyspnea is an unpleasant awareness of difficult breathing and has been the

subject of considerable interest and extensive investigation for a great many years. The neurophysiological basis for the symptom is not completely understood, but it is likely that stretch receptors in the respiratory muscles signal the discomfort associated with excessive respiratory work. The increased work of breathing is due either to restriction of lung or chest, making it difficult to expand the lungs, or to obstruction of the flow of air into and out of the lung. In many patients, hyperventilation, induced by excessive reflex stimulation to breathing, adds to the respiratory work and sense of discomfort. This is particularly true in pulmonary congestion and diffuse interstitial lung disease, in which the hyperventilation of a stiff lung is the major cause of dyspnea. In pulmonary embolism the reflex hyperventilation causes dyspnea even in the absence of abnormal lung mechanics.

In evaluating the patient with dyspnea, it is important to remember that, even in heart disease, the symptom is due to abnormal pulmonary mechanics and that similar derangements may be present in pulmonary congestion due to ventricular failure as in obstructive or restrictive lung disease. Unfortunately, the symptom does not appear to be particularly different in the wide range of conditions that cause it, and the physician must seek to understand the nature and the cause of impeded breathing. Spirometry is an essential step in evaluating the patient with dyspnea in order to learn whether obstructive or restrictive lung disease is present in sufficient degree to account for the complaint.

Dyspnea, usually with cough, is frequently a major complaint in patients with pulmonary infection, both chronic and acute, and it may be an important symptom in a wide variety of systemic illnesses. Usually these conditions are self-evident and infections, such as tuberculosis, are always associated with abnormalities of the x-ray film of the chest if of sufficient severity to cause shortness of breath.

When dyspnea is the dominant symptom, a number of conditions must be considered. In left ventricular failure, the shortness of breath is due to exudation of fluid, making the lung stiffer than normal. In addition, fluid tends to track up along the airways, causing obstruction to air flow, and the distended capillaries cause reflex hyperventilation. Dyspnea usually develops gradually over a long period of time and is associated with a readily detectable abnormality of the heart. X-ray film of the chest reveals vascular

Table 1–1 Dyspnea: A Spirometric Classification

Obstructive Disease
  Asthma
  COPD
  Pulmonary congestion
  Upper airway obstruction

Restrictive Disease
  Diffuse lung disease
  Spontaneous pneumothorax
  Pulmonary congestion

Normal Spirogram
  Pulmonary embolism
  Anxiety

redistribution from the lower to upper lobes and, in more advanced cases, alveolar infiltrates. Late inspiratory crackles are audible at the bases of the lungs, but these are identical to the sounds that may be present in diffuse interstitial lung disease. Indeed, diffuse lung disease, considered in more detail in Chapter 5, produces effects on pulmonary function similar to those of pulmonary congestion, namely stiffening of the lungs with reduction of vital capacity. The x-ray film of the chest may be similar in the two conditions, but pulmonary congestion is more apt to be associated with a large heart, vascular redistribution, and less discrete fibronodular infiltrates. However, there are exceptions, and diffuse lung disease may not cause severe abnormality of the roentgenogram, so that the distinction may be difficult. A very useful test under these circumstances is measurement of the diffusing capacity for carbon monoxide. In interstitial disease this capacity is always below normal, whereas in pulmonary congestion it may be normal or even elevated because of the increased volume of the pulmonary capillary bed resulting from increase in left atrial pressure.

Pulmonary congestion due to left ventricular failure may also be associated with airway obstruction, sometimes even manifest as wheeze (cardiac asthma). It is important to obtain an adequate history, particularly of ischemic heart disease, and to search for other physical and radiographic evidence of cardiac abnormality. Asthma, discussed in detail in Chapter 2, is much more variable than the progressive shortness of breath associated with heart disease, and patients with asthma almost always have a characteristic sensation of tightness and, usually, measurable improvement of expiratory flow rate after administration of bronchodilators. Chronic obstructive pulmonary disease may be slowly progressive in nature but is almost always associated with cough, and the heart is normal and often of small size. The features distinguishing nocturnal dyspnea from the worsening of symptoms experienced when the patient with obstructive disease lies down have been noted under Cough.

In most of these conditions the nature of the chronic illness is known to the patient and the physician, but sometimes it is necessary to consider left ventricular failure as a new complication in a patient with chronic respiratory distress due to obstructive or restrictive lung disease. This should be reflected in cardiac enlargement and pulmonary vascular changes, but it may be necessary to give a therapeutic trial of cardiotonic agents. If diuretic therapy is associated with substantial increase of vital capacity, one may conclude that pulmonary congestion is an important component of the patient's shortness of breath.

There are a number of other conditions in which dyspnea is the main complaint. Upper airway obstruction, discussed in more detail in Chapter 10, is generally associated with audible stridor over the trachea; and spontaneous pneumothorax, not always evident on physical examination, is clearly revealed by chest roentgenogram. Pulmonary embolism, discussed in Chapter 8, is a common cause of dyspnea, and it may not be associated with abnormalities on physical or x-ray examination. It is extremely important to search for predisposing causes, to examine the legs carefully, and to measure arterial blood gas tensions. Significant pulmonary embolization should be associated with widening of the alveolar arterial oxygen gradient. In some patients, pulmonary embolism is likely to be confused with anxiety, but the latter is more commonly associated with an inability to get a deep breath rather than true shortness of breath. In anxiety states, respirations are apt to be irregular, with sighs and yawns rather than the rapid shallow breathing characteristic of embolism. In doubtful cases, an increase in the A-a oxygen gradient strongly favors embolism, and a lung scan may be extremely useful.

Pericardial tamponade may be associated with severe dyspnea, particularly when the patient lies down, because of compression of the pulmonary veins behind the heart. The diagnosis is usually suggested by radiographic evidence of an enlarged cardiac silhouette and is most quickly and easily confirmed by echocardiography.

Other Symptoms

Other important symptoms of pulmonary disease include chest pain and fever. Chest pain is usually the result of inflammation of sensory nerves in the pleura. It is characteristically worse with breathing and coughing. Some patients with carcinoma of the lung complain of discomfort, though the source of this pain is not entirely clear. Tumors that invade the chest wall characteristically produce pain, often with involvement of nerve roots, and this must be defined and evaluated. Pulmonary hypertension is associated with chest pain not unlike that of angina pectoris, though usually it is higher in location and not relieved by nitroglycerin. It may be induced by exertion, described as crushing, and relieved by rest.

Noisy breathing is another symptom often evident to the patient. Wheezing is particularly common in asthma and is generally polyphonic and variable. The presence of a localized, persistent rhonchus or wheeze strongly suggests fixed airway obstruction, as from a tumor. Upper airway obstruction, particularly during sleep, is being recognized with increasing frequency (sleep apnea syndrome). It is particularly common in obesity but not confined to patients who are overweight. Patients with this problem may present with excessive somnolence during the day and even cor pulmonale. The first clue may be a history of loud snoring associated with periodic interruption of sleep. Usually the spouse or other family members can supply a better history of loud snoring and apnea interrupting the sleep through the night. A stridor or wheeze in the larynx may be the result of tracheal compression or stenosis.

Other Important Information

An occupational history is particularly important in patients with pulmonary disease, and *all* occupations should be described in as much detail as possible. One must be concerned about the development of lung cancer in patients exposed to asbestos. A wide variety of dusts and chemicals are known to cause interstitial disease of the lung, and asthma may result from a great many chemicals both in nature and industry. Other types of allergic lung disease have resulted from exposure to molds growing in air-conditioners. A careful history of drug ingestion is equally important, since a number of drugs have recently been incriminated in a range of diseases, from pulmonary edema to diffuse interstitial lung disease. Oily nose drops or nocturnal use of mineral oil may be the clue to the presence of lipid pneumonia; aspirin may be an important cause of asthma in many patients.

One should know the various areas in which the patient has lived, particularly in reference to the possibility of fungal infections with limited geographic localization. The patient with acute respiratory illness is more likely to have a mycoplasmic than bacterial infection if other members of the family or community have recently been infected. Ornithosis must be considered in the patient who is devoted to parrots, parakeets, pigeons, or ducks. One of the most important aspects of history taking is careful inquiry into personal habits. A detailed smoking history is particularly important, including the type and amount of material smoked and whether or not inhaled. The risk of lung cancer, bronchitis, and emphysema is practically negligible in nonsmokers, although the slow rate of growth of a tumor from its initial appearance means that many years must pass before the exsmoker is out of danger. Smoking impairs mucociliary clearance and, probably, macrophage function, so that it may predispose to pulmonary infection and almost certainly to postoperative complications. The history represents the physician's first opportunity to educate the patient about smoking and, it is hoped, to persuade the patient to give it up.

Other habits are important. Alcohol also impairs mucociliary clearance and pulmonary defenses, predisposing the user to pulmonary infections and chronic lung disease. So does heroin. Chronic lung disease, particularly emphysema, is common in addicts. Bronchiectasis has been reported to be extremely common after heroin pulmonary edema. An intravenous drug user is susceptible to septic pulmonary embolism, and this serious condition, perhaps associated with endocarditis, must be considered in an addict with fever and multiple pulmonary infiltrates, particularly if they contain cavities.

Associated systemic symptoms are important, since a wide variety of infectious and noninfectious diseases, ranging from tuberculosis and fungal infection to collagen vascular disease, are apt to involve both the lungs and other organs. A previous history of pneumonia, particularly if recurrent and in the same location, strongly suggests the presence of chronic underlying bronchial disease, such as bronchiectasis, or even a neoplasm. Pneumonia or whooping cough in childhood may cause bronchiectasis that does not become symptomatic until adult life, and there is now evidence that the smoker who experienced any childhood respiratory illness is particularly at risk of developing chronic obstructive pulmonary disease.

In patients with chronic illness it is extremely important to get a sense of the tempo and rate of development of the illness. Diffuse interstitial lung disease that develops relatively acutely is much more apt to respond satisfactorily to corticosteroids than is the slowly progressive, indolent interstitial fibrosis. In sarcoidosis, most of the symptoms develop within the first year, and the development of new symptoms suggests an additional or alternative diagnosis.

In obtaining a history the physician should pay attention to the emotional state of the patient. The intensity of symptoms must be evaluated in the light of the patient's tendency to exaggerate or to minimize complaints. Sometimes the nature of the description can lead to a diagnosis of hyperventilation as the cause of dyspnea. Certainly the severity of asthma is closely related to the patient's emotional state, and careful inquiry is needed to clarify important precipitants of this condition. Many diseases may be related to attitudes, fears, and moods. There is evidence that tuberculosis is apt to develop after a serious emotional deprivation, and people who respond to sorrow by giving up are probably more apt to get ill with this and other diseases than those who cope more actively and successfully. This is but a glimpse into how life's events and their effect on the patient may have bearing on the development of pulmonary disease. Inquiry of this sort not only provides demonstrable evidence to the patient of the physician's empathy and interest, but it adds an additional dimension to the physician's understanding of health and disease.

PHYSICAL EXAMINATION

Although x-ray and pulmonary function examinations have added remarkable precision to our evaluation of patients, and they are essential, useful information can be obtained from the physical examination, some of it not evident in any other way. In addition, like history taking, performance of a physical examination serves an important therapeutic function in enhancing the patient-physician relationship. One experienced physician has pointed out that there is nothing like a good "mauling" to break down the barriers between patient and physician.

Respiratory Movements

A great deal of information can be obtained by careful observation of respiratory movements. Pursed-lips breathing, intuitively adopted by patients with chronic obstructive pulmonary disease to prevent expiratory collapse of airways, is virtually diagnostic. The barrel chest of emphysema may be more a reflection of abdominal wasting than lung overinflation, but there are other findings that are useful in evaluating obstructive airway disease. With severe airway obstruction, the normal bucket handle motion of the ribs is lost; lateral expansion of the chest cage is diminished, and the lower intercostal margins retract rather than expand with inspiration (Hoover's sign). Lack of diaphragmatic function is reflected in absent protrusion of the abdomen during inspiration, and in respiratory failure there is even paradoxical retraction of the abdominal wall, suggesting elevation of the diaphragm during inspiration. Severe airway obstruction requires use of the accessory muscles of respiration, and palpable tensing of the scalenus and sternocleidomastoid muscles is a useful indication of severe obstructive airway disease, including asthma. The presence and extent of airway obstruction can be evaluated by listening to a forced expiration over the trachea. After a full inspiration, expiration is normally complete within three seconds, and the degree of prolongation reflects the severity of obstruction. None of these tests has the precision and accuracy of spirometric study, but they do provide a useful starting point.

It is important to observe the pattern of breathing. Diffuse lung disease is characterized by rapid shallow respirations; patients with anxiety are apt to breathe irregularly with frequent sighs; and abnormal breathing patterns, such as Cheyne Stokes respiration, signify serious congestive heart failure or neurological disturbance. Occasionally it is possible to detect diaphragmatic paralysis by unilateral expansion of the abdomen during inspiration. Upper airway obstruction, by either a mass or tracheal narrowing, is detected by the presence of a stridor during forced inspiration and expiration over the trachea.

Examination of the Lungs

Systematic percussion and auscultation of the chest continue to play an important role in the examination of patients. Dullness to percussion may indicate the presence of pleural effusion or of consolidation, but this is far less reliable than the x-ray film of the chest. Normal breath sounds are generated by movement of air through the large airways and increased or decreased transmission of these sounds signifies the presence of intervening fluid, tissue, or air in the lung or pleura between the source of the sounds and the stethoscope. A consolidated lung or, on occasion, a pleural effusion transmits bronchial sounds to the chest. Overinflation of the lungs, obstructed airways, pleural thickening, effusion, and pneumothorax cause reduction of the breath sounds.

Adventitious sounds are extremely important, and in recent years they have generated new interest and attempts at standardization and simplification. These sounds are now divided into discontinuous and continuous sounds. Discontinuous sounds, previously called rales, and now preferably termed crackles, are the interrupted, explosive sounds usually heard during inspiration. Some feel that they can be subdivided into coarse and fine crackles. The former are more common in pulmonary edema or pneumonia; the latter, in diffuse interstitial lung disease. In both cases, the sounds probably result from the explosive opening of small airways that collapsed during the previous expiration, and it may be very difficult indeed to distinguish between the crackles of pulmonary edema and interstitial fibrosis. Inspiratory crackles are much more common in interstitial fibrosis and pneumoconiosis than in the diffuse lung disease associated with sarcoidosis or other types of granuloma. Crackles are also heard in obstructive pulmonary disease, but they occur early rather than late during inspiration and may also be associated with expiratory sounds, presumably resulting from abrupt changes of the caliber of airways during expiration as well as inspiration. Continuous sounds are subdivided into wheezes and rhonchi, the former being a high-pitched musical sound and the latter being lower pitched and sonorous. These findings reflect variable narrowing of the airways, though they are not discriminatory with respect to site or nature of airway obstruction. It is true that musical wheezes are characteristic of asthma, but they may be heard in other types of obstructive disease and they may be absent in asthma. They do not reflect the severity of the obstruction. A localized, single rhonchus is a very important finding, suggesting fixed airway obstruction, as from a tumor. Since this may be palpable but not audible, it is wise for the physician to perform bimanual palpation over the different areas of the thorax during a forced inspiration and expiration.

Other adventitious sounds include the leathery, to and fro friction rub synchronous with the heart beat or respiration and indicative of pericarditis or pleurisy, respectively, and the systolic crunching sound associated with mediastinal emphysema.

Other Findings

Careful examination of the neck may be very revealing. Palpation of the trachea to determine whether or not it is deviated is best accomplished by placing the thumb in the suprasternal notch. Occasionally tracheal deviation can be noted in this fashion when it is not evident on x-ray. Palpable supraclavicular nodes, felt by deep compression in the supraclavicular space, aided by compression of soft tissue below the clavicle into the examining finger, may reveal lymph nodes containing tumor or sarcoid granuloma, which can be proven by biopsy. Crepitus in the neck is an important sign of pneumomediastinum, which may or may not accompany pneumothorax, and the presence of Horner's syndrome may signify a superior sulcus tumor. Venous distention of the neck is an important sign of right-sided heart failure or of superior vena cava obstruction from carcinoma of the lung.

Clubbing of the fingers is a very important finding in pulmonary disease. At an early stage, it may only be evident as loss of the nail-nailbed angle and as sponginess of the nailbed. It may be the only or initial manifestation of lung cancer, or it may indicate the presence of suppurative disease such as lung abscess or bronchiectasis. Cyanosis of the nailbeds is a very inaccurate and insensitive indication of hypoxemia; but if present, it indicates a need for arterial blood gas analysis. Telangiectases on the skin or lips suggest that a lung lesion, particularly in a patient with hemoptysis, is a pulmonary arteriovenous fistula. There are a variety of other skin findings of importance, including erythema nodosum, which when coupled with asymptomatic hilar adenopathy, may be sufficient to make a diagnosis of sarcoidosis, and the occasional metastatic skin nodule may obviate the need for deeper biopsy. Physical findings of rheumatoid arthritis are very important because rheumatoid disease is not only associated with pleural effusion but may cause obliterative airway disease or nodular infiltrates in the lung. Other types of collagen vascular disease, particularly scleroderma, are often associated with pulmonary infiltrates and pulmonary fibrosis.

SPUTUM EXAMINATION

Examination of expectorated sputum is a very important step in all patients with any degree of cough. It is important that the specimen represent material originating in the tracheobronchial tree rather than saliva and that the patient cough and expectorate directly into an appropriate container. Sputum production may be induced by inhalation of heated hypertonic aerosols or, in acutely ill patients, by transtracheal aspiration or even fibroptic bronchoscopy. Because there is a significant risk of complications, transtracheal aspiration should only be performed by an experienced physician, and obviously bronchoscopy requires specialized skill and training. It is important to observe the odor and the character of the sputum, particularly for the presence of blood, and material must be sent for cultures, including cultures for tubercle bacilli and fungi and for cytology in patients with chronic cough.

The immediate examination should include both a gram stain and Wright stain. A gram stain will reveal a preponderance of a single type of bacteria in most cases of acute bacterial infection, and this becomes the preliminary guide to therapy with appropriate antibiotics. One should only pay attention to real sputum, as evidenced by the presence of polymorpho-nuclear leukocytes, macrophages, and bronchial cells and the relative absence of buccal epithelial cells. Wright's stain is useful in revealing a proponderance of eosinophils, suggestive of asthma or asthmatic bronchitis.

X-RAY

A posteroanterior (PA) x-ray film of the chest is an essential component of the pulmonary workup. Any patient with pulmonary symptoms or fever requires such an examination. More definitive detail and localization will be provided by lateral and oblique views, and an apical lordotic film may reveal a lesion hidden under the clavicle on the PA film. If there is symptomatic or physical evidence of pleurisy, one should also order decubitus films in order to reveal a small pleural effusion that may not be otherwise evident. It has been shown that a substantial number of patients with mycoplasma pneumonia have pleural effusion that is evident only in the decubitus position.

In some patients a PA film taken during inspiration and expiration can be very useful. Such a study may reveal abnormal motion of one diaphragm, which is best evaluated by fluoroscopy, or may better outline an air pocket, as in a bulla or pneumothorax.

X-ray examination is most useful in delineating solid lesions in the lung. It is of far less value in obstructive pulmonary disease. Patients with both bronchitis and asthma have thickening of the walls of the airways, but these findings are nonspecific and of little diagnostic value, as is the hyperinflation of the lung encountered in all types of obstructing pulmonary disease. This type of pathology is much better delineated by pulmonary function studies, but tomograms and angiograms are useful for outlining the location and extent of emphysema. Radiographic studies are very helpful in suggesting the nature of diffuse lung disease, which is usefully subdivided into alveolar filling disease, characterized by the presence of an air bronchogram and fluffy diffuse infiltrates, and interstitial disease of the lung in which reticular-nodular lesions are scattered throughout the parenchyma, often with a honeycomb appearance. The roentgenogram is also a very sensitive indicator of pulmonary congestion. In this condition the vessels in the upper lobes become more prominent than those in the lower lobe (vascular redistribution), and their outlines become fluffy and irregular because of the presence of perivascular fluid. These changes may be present before any other signs of pulmonary congestion, including crackles.

Tomographic Studies

Tomographic studies are indicated for precise delineation of radiographic lesions such as cavitation or when one wishes to ascertain whether or not other lesions are present. Tomograms are particularly useful in the evaluation of patients with coin lesions to search for calcification, to delineate the margins of the lesion, and to reveal the presence of additional nodules that might represent metastasis. Tomograms may also reveal the details of airway structure in a patient with pneumonic consolidation, suggesting the need for bronchoscopy if the major airways are abnormal. Patients with unresolved pneumonia or with recurrent pneumonia in the same area should have such a study.

Bronchography

Bronchography requires the introduction of contrast material into the tracheobronchial tree and is primarily used for evaluation of patients with bronchiectasis. If a patient is to have surgery for bronchiectasis, a bronchogram is necessary to outline the extent of the disease. This evaluation is now performed infrequently, since surgery, except in cases of major hemoptysis, has largely been replaced by medical therapy. Bronchography may also reveal an obstructing tumor not evident on other films, but this indication for the examination has also declined greatly, since the fiberoptic bronchoscope provides direct access to the smaller airways.

Perfusion Scans

Perfusion scans are mainly useful if the PA film of the chest is normal. Perfusion defects in patients with otherwise normal lungs are strongly suggestive of pulmonary embolism, particularly if a ventilation scan is normal, indicating an isolated abnormality of the circulation.

Angiography

It is now felt, however, that definitive diagnosis of pulmonary embolism requires angiography. This examination is most commonly performed in patients in whom pulmonary embolism is suspected, but it is also used for the evaluation of patients with carcinoma of the lung in a search for invasion of central vascular structures.

Barium Swallow

A barium swallow is an important screening procedure for mediastinal involvement in patients with lung cancer and is also useful in searching for lesions that might cause recurrent aspiration pneumonia.

PULMONARY FUNCTION STUDIES

Spirometry and Expiratory Flow Rates

Most of the tests of pulmonary function that are needed for the evaluation of the pulmonary patient can be performed by the physician in his office.

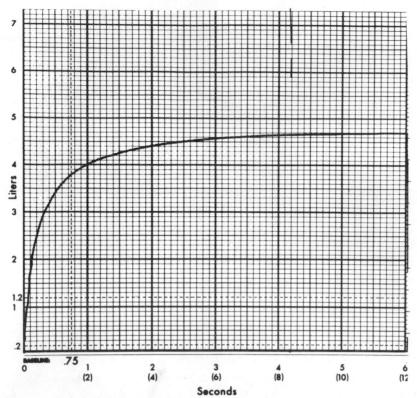

Figure 1-1 Spirometric tracing obtained from a normal young man. The vital capacity is 4.7 liters, 97 per cent is expired in 3 seconds (FEV_1/FEV_3), and one second volume, FEV_1, is 4.0 liters. (This and the following three figures were kindly supplied by Thomas L. Petty, M.D., University of Colorado Medical Center).

Spirometric testing should be just as much a part of the evaluation of the patient with lung disease as an electrocardiogram is a part of the workup of the patient with heart disease. Spirometry is performed by having patients fill their lungs and then expire as hard and as fast as possible into a recording spirometer. Simple, small spirometers are now available at a relatively modest cost. From the spirometric tracing, the physician should calculate the volume of the vital capacity (VC), the volume and percentage expired in the first second (FEV_1 and FEV_1/VC, respectively) and the maximal mid-expiratory flow rate, FEF25–75%. This will provide the critical information for evaluating the patient with either obstructive or restrictive disease of the lung.

Obstructive disease is characterized by slowing of the forced expiration, with reduced FEV_1, FEV_1/VC, and FEF25-75%. This is often accompanied by reduction of vital capacity because of closure of airways, but flow rates are reduced more. Restrictive disease, from either diffuse interstitial lung disease or extensive consolidation of the lung from infection or tumor, is characterized by reduction of vital capacity without slowing of the forced expiratory rate. Spirometry is absolutely essential for evaluation of the patient with dyspnea, for an estimation of the severity of the disease, and for following its progress. Response to treatment provides extremely important information. In congestive failure, effective therapy should be accompanied by improved vital capacity, and this may be of diagnostic value in puzzling cases. In sarcoidosis, one indication for corticosteroid therapy is severe impairment of lung function, and the vital capacity is an important guide to steroid dosage. The value of corticosteroids to a patient with obstructive lung disease should be documented by improved expiratory flow rates. In patients with obstructive lung disease, the spirogram should be repeated 10 minutes after inhalation of a bronchodilating aerosol in order to assess the extent of reversibility. The test may have to be repeated many times before one can make a diagnosis of irreversible lung disease.

An annual spirometric examination is just as important for the smoker, who is at risk of developing obstructive lung disease as well as lung cancer, as an x-ray film of the chest. Rapid deterioration of FEV_1 may provide warning that chronic obstructive pulmonary disease is developing, just as the chest roentgenogram may reveal a tumor before symptoms appear. It is important to add, however, that even semiannual chest roentgenograms do not, in the majority of instances, reveal a diagnosis of lung cancer at an early enough stage to permit successful surgery.

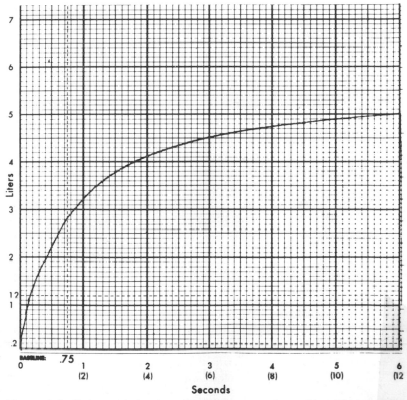

Figure 1–2 Spirometric tracing obtained from a patient with mild obstructive pulmonary disease. Although the vital capacity is normal, the FEV_1 of 3.2 liters is slightly below predicted and there is continuing expiration after 3 seconds.

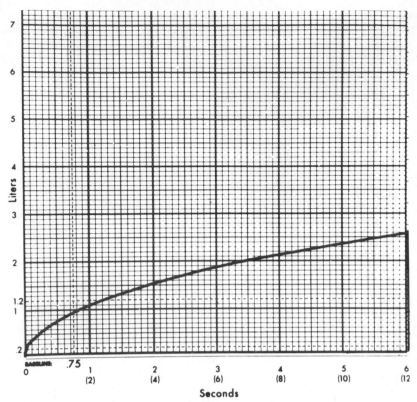

Figure 1–3 Spirometric tracing obtained from a patient with severe obstructive pulmonary disease with pronounced slowing throughout the entire expiration and substantial reduction of vital capacity.

One other test is particularly useful in chest medicine and that is the measurement of the peak expiratory flow rate by a small, portable meter, which can be kept by patients for their own use or carried by the physician to ward or bedside.* This measurement is particularly useful in evaluating the severity of asthma and, as will be discussed in Chapter 2, should be part of each examination of the patient with asthma in order to assess the severity of the condition and the response to therapy.

Arterial Blood Gases

Arterial blood gas analysis is rarely needed for the assessment of outpatients but is indicated in most patients hospitalized with severe pulmonary disease and in patients with symptomatic dyspnea or extensive involvement on roentgenogram. Hypoxemia, which may require therapy, can only be detected with accuracy by arterial blood gas analysis. Assessment of the adequacy of alveolar ventilation and the need for ventilatory support or

---

*Mini Wright Peak Flow Meter, Armstrong Industries, Inc., P.O. Box 7, 3660 Commercial Avenue, Northbrook, Illinois 60062 (800-323-4220).

intensive respiratory care can only be provided by measurement of the arterial P_{CO_2}. The physician must have a working familiarity with the meaning of arterial blood gas measurements, and this will be discussed further in Chapter 9.

Specialized Tests of Pulmonary Function

Almost all of the information that is important to the practicing physician in the evaluation and treatment of patients with pulmonary disease can be obtained from spirometry and analysis of arterial blood gas composition. However, there are a great many other tests of pulmonary function that are very important to our understanding of pulmonary disease and its development and, on occasion, they may be of practical benefit. These tests will be described briefly, with emphasis on the information that they provide that is useful in clinical medicine.

Lung Volume

Measurements of lung volume reveal the amount of air contained in the lung at a designated volume, generally functional residual capacity (FRC) or total

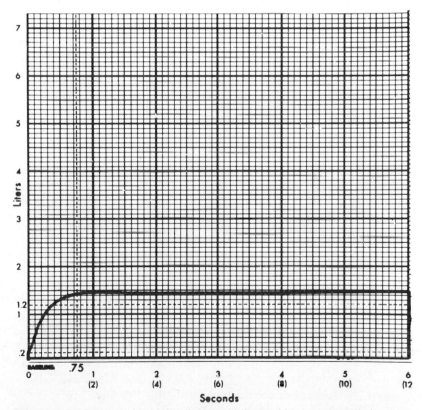

Figure 1–4 Spirometric tracing from a patient with severe restrictive lung disease with marked reduction of vital capacity, which is entirely expelled within the first second.

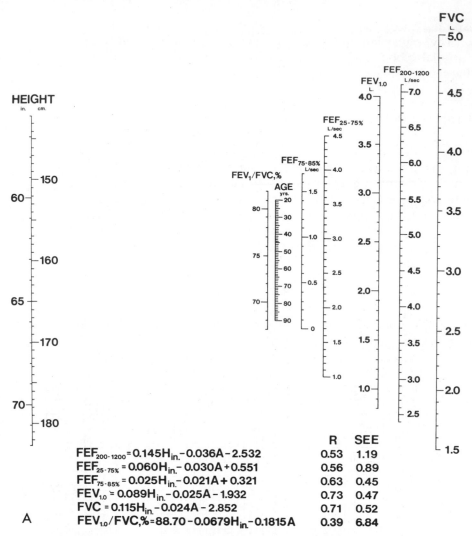

	R	SEE
$FEF_{200-1200} = 0.145H_{in.} - 0.036A - 2.532$	0.53	1.19
$FEF_{25-75\%} = 0.060H_{in.} - 0.030A + 0.551$	0.56	0.89
$FEF_{75-85\%} = 0.025H_{in.} - 0.021A + 0.321$	0.63	0.45
$FEV_{1.0} = 0.089H_{in.} - 0.025A - 1.932$	0.73	0.47
$FVC = 0.115H_{in.} - 0.024A - 2.852$	0.71	0.52
$FEV_{1.0}/FVC,\% = 88.70 - 0.0679H_{in.} - 0.1815A$	0.39	6.84

Figure 1–5 Pulmonary function standards for normal females *(A)* and males *(B)*. To use the nomogram, lay a straightedge between the patient's height as read on the HEIGHT scale and his or her age as it appears on the AGE scale. (From Morris, J. F.: Spirometry in evaluation of pulmonary function. West. J. Med., *125*:114–115, 1976.)

illustration continued on opposite page

lung capacity (TLC). The FRC can be obtained by determining the degree to which an inert gas, of known concentration and volume, is diluted by the air within the lung. This technique has the disadvantage of not measuring the amount of air contained in nonventilated or very poorly ventilated units of lung, so that it may underestimate the true volume. Body plethysmography reveals the total amount of air in the lung, regardless of ventilation, and radiographic techniques, utilizing PA and lateral x-ray films of the chest, provide a relatively simple, inexpensive, and accurate method for measuring the TLC and FRC.

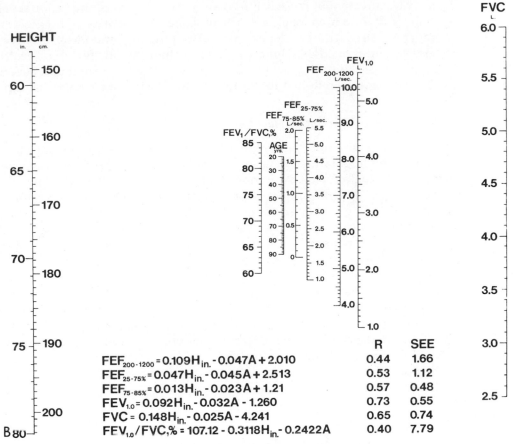

$$FEF_{200\text{-}1200} = 0.109H_{in.} - 0.047A + 2.010 \qquad 0.44 \quad 1.66$$
$$FEF_{25\text{-}75\%} = 0.047H_{in.} - 0.045A + 2.513 \qquad 0.53 \quad 1.12$$
$$FEF_{75\text{-}85\%} = 0.013H_{in.} - 0.023A + 1.21 \qquad 0.57 \quad 0.48$$
$$FEV_{1.0} = 0.092H_{in.} - 0.032A - 1.260 \qquad 0.73 \quad 0.55$$
$$FVC = 0.148H_{in.} - 0.025A - 4.241 \qquad 0.65 \quad 0.74$$
$$FEV_{1.0}/FVC,\% = 107.12 - 0.3118H_{in.} - 0.2422A \qquad 0.40 \quad 7.79$$

R   SEE

Figure 1–5 *Continued*

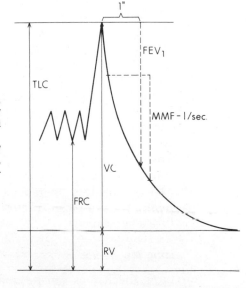

Figure 1–6 Schematic representation of lung volumes, total lung capacity (TLC), functional residual capacity (FRC), vital capacity (VC), residual volume (RV), and of a forced expiration depicting forced expiratory volume in one second (FEV₁), and maximum mid-expiratory flow rate (MMF). (From Beeson, Paul B., and McDermott, Walsh (eds.): Textbook of Medicine. 14th edition. Philadelphia, W. B. Saunders Company, 1975.)

Measurement of these volumes, and, by derivation, the residual volume (RV), is of little functional or practical value. An increase of lung volume is generally a reflection of the severity of emphysema and of obstructive lung disease and reduction of lung volume is a characteristic feature of restrictive lung disease. But the practical information about the extent and severity of these diseases is reflected in the spirometric tracing of a forced vital capacity.

Inspiratory and Expiratory Flow Rates

Recording inspiratory and expiratory flow rates in relationship to the lung volume highlights the characteristic reduction of expiratory flow rate that occurs during a forced expiration, and measurement of flow rate at a given volume by this technique is one means of quantifying expiratory flow limitation. The expiratory flow rate at low lung volumes is a particularly sensitive indicator of small airway disease. At one time it was thought that a characteristic pattern of flow rate in relation to volume might distinguish between different types of obstructive lung disease, but this apparently is not the case. Furthermore, the same information can be obtained from careful spirometric tracings, and there is little practical advantage to the use of this technique. However, recording of inspiratory flow rate is important in assessing the presence of a fixed obstruction of the airways either within or outside of the chest, since more reduction of inspiratory than expiratory flow is characteristic of such a lesion. Once again, however, this information can be obtained from spirometry, if one measures a forced inspiration as well as the forced expiratory vital capacity.

Diffusing Capacity

The diffusing capacity of the lung is a reflection of the area and thinness of the alveolar capillary membrane involved in the diffusion of gases within the lung. Reduction of the diffusing capacity is a characteristic feature of emphysema, because of loss of the surface area available for diffusion, and of interstitial lung diseases, such as diffuse interstitial fibrosis or sarcoidosis. In emphysema, the extent of the disease is reflected in the degree of reduction of diffusing capacity, but this is of little practical importance for the management of patients. In pulmonary fibrosis, the reduction of diffusing capacity correlates fairly well with the reduction of vital capacity and there is little need to study diffusion as well as vital capacity in evaluating and treating patients with this group of disorders. In recent years, there has been some interest in the fact that hemorrhage into the lung may be reflected in an increase of the diffusing capacity. This results from the high affinity of carbon monoxide, the gas used for measuring diffusion, for red blood cells whether they are located in alveolar capillaries or in the alveoli themselves. Thus, this measurement may be of some value in following patients with intrapulmonary hemorrhage in order to ascertain the severity of the process and to consider therapeutic intervention, such as surgery for localized hemoptysis or plasmapheresis for the hemorrhage associated with Goodpasture's syndrome.

Lung Mechanics

Lung mechanics can be quantified accurately either by body plethysmography or by simultaneous measurement of intrapleural pressure, reflected in the pressure measured by a tube placed in the esophagus, and inspiratory and expiratory flow rates. The latter permits calculation both of airway resistance and of lung compliance. In general, an increase in airway resistance is reflected in reduction of expiratory flow rates. The site or nature of pathology is not revealed by this measurement any more than it is by spirometry. Lung compliance is reduced, or the lungs become stiffer, in diffuse interstitial lung disease, but this too is reflected in reduction of the vital capacity. Increase of lung compliance appears to be a fairly accurate indicator of the extent of emphysema, as is reduction of diffusing capacity, but this information is more of interest than of importance to the management of the patient.

Small Airways Disease

A great many techniques have been developed for the study of small airways disease. These include frequency dependence of compliance, closing volume, expiratory flow rates at low lung volumes, and studies of gas mixing within the lung. Frequency dependence of compliance refers to the fact that the presence of nonuniform obstruction of small airways causes the measured compliance to fall as respiratory frequency is increased. This is due to the fact that, at rapid frequencies, the obstructed airways do not become ventilated, causing a reduction in the total amount of ventilated lung and, hence, a fall in compliance. Closing volume refers to the fact that, as the lung empties, partially obstructed airways may close completely, so that the alveoli they ventilate no longer empty, leading to a change in the concentration of expired gas. Flow rates at low lung volumes are discussed under Inspiratory and Expiratory Flow Rates. Uneven gas mixing will occur when there is a variable degree of obstruction of small airways, and this is reflected in the changing concentration of a foreign gas during a forced expiration.

All of these measurements provide sensitive indications of small airways disease, which may be present in the absence of any symptoms at all. As a result, they may detect abnormalities in the lung in people, particularly smokers, who are perfectly healthy. It is possible that patients with such an abnormality are those who will go on to develop obstructive lung disease in the years to come. However, this has not been proven to be the case; and since, aside from discontinuing smoking, there is little that can be done to prevent obstructive lung disease, these tests cannot be recommended for individual patients. They are, however, of great value in long-term studies of populations and in epidemiological studies to determine the prevalence of disease in groups of people exposed to various air pollutants.

Ventilation/Perfusion Abnormalities

Ventilation/perfusion ($\dot{V}/\dot{Q}$) abnormalities are the dominant causes of hypoxemia in patients with pulmonary disease. $\dot{V}/\dot{Q}$ abnormality refers to the fact that some units of lung are perfused more than they are ventilated or ventilated more than they are perfused. The result is hypoxemia, predominantly related to the perfusion of poorly ventilated units, and an increase of the physiological dead space, predominantly a reflection of ventilation of poorly perfused areas of lung. These abnormalities are quantified in a variety of ways, including radioisotope techniques for actually measuring $\dot{V}/\dot{Q}$ ratios in different parts of the lung, measurement of physiological dead space, and measurement of the alveolar arterial oxygen tension gradient, the difference between the partial pressure of oxygen in the alveolar air and in arterial blood. Once again, these measurements add a great deal of precision to our understanding of pulmonary disease and its effect on lung function, but they add little to our treatment of the patient. The end point of treatment of hypoxemia is an increase of arterial oxygen tension, generally by the administration of increased amounts of inspired oxygen, and this is reflected in measurements of arterial Po_2. Increase of physiological dead space requires increased amounts of ventilation, as in patients on a respirator, but the criterion of such therapy is, again, the simple measurement of arterial Pco_2.

Right-to-Left Shunt

An extreme form of $\dot{V}/\dot{Q}$ disturbance is a right-to-left shunt, which occurs when blood perfuses alveoli that are totally nonventilated. This occurs in atelectasis, although perfusion is greatly decreased in the collapsed lung, in pulmonary edema, when the fluid-filled alveoli cannot be ventilated, and in arteriovenous fistula. Detection of such shunts is easily made by measuring the arterial Po_2 during 100 per cent oxygen breathing. Under these circumstances any decrease of Po_2 below the expected value can be ascribed to shunting, and the size of the shunt can be calculated. Such measurement is of value in treating patients with various types of pulmonary edema (Chapter 9) and may be of diagnostic value in establishing the cause of hypoxemia.

Respiratory Control

Disturbance of respiratory control may be an important cause of hypoventilation, particularly in patients with obstructive lung disease and, rarely, in patients with normal lungs (Chapter 9). The respiratory control system can be evaluated by measuring the increase of minute ventilation caused by inspiring increasing concentrations of carbon dioxide or decreasing concentrations of oxygen, testing the two chemoreceptor systems. More accurately, evaluation can be achieved by studying respiratory muscle force, the pressure generated by respiratory muscles under these conditions. This eliminates the effects of abnormal lung mechanics on the respiratory response to hypercapnia and hypoxemia. Once again, studies such as this have shed a great deal of light on abnormalities of respiratory control in a variety of pulmonary diseases, particularly the hypoventilation associated with obesity, but they are of little value in diagnosis and treatment.

A major exception is the rare patient with primary alveolar hypoventilation, apparently an isolated defect of the respiratory center that causes hypoventilation and hypercapnia in the presence of normal lungs and chest wall (Chapter 9). The diagnosis of this condition is made with certainty by demonstrating complete absence of the ventilatory response to inhaled carbon dioxide. It is possible that individuals with a hypoactive response to carbon dioxide will be the people who develop hypoventilation when they acquire other illness such as obstructive lung disease or obesity, and it is possible that there is an important genetic component to the sudden infant death syndrome, which would be reflected in reduced respiratory response in parents of children destined to experience this sudden, fatal disorder. However, these relationships remain to be proven. Even if true, it is not clear that screening of relatives or of individuals would be an important practical measure for the prevention or control of pulmonary disease.

SPECIALIZED DIAGNOSTIC PROCEDURES

Bronchofiberscopy

The development of relatively small, flexible bronchoscopes that permit access to airways not accessible to the rigid bronchoscope and that can be introduced in the conscious patient with little discomfort or hazard has added enormously to our ability to make a precise diagnosis in a wide variety of pulmonary diseases. Fiberoptic bronchoscopy can only be performed by a trained, experienced physician, but the indications and value of the examination, as well as the risks and limitations, should be understood by the practicing physician. The bronchofiberscope permits inspection of the upper airways and then the major bronchi, for detection of compressing lesions or abnormalities, ranging from foreign body occlusion of a segmental bronchus to bronchial tumors. Forceps permit biopsy of visible lesions for accurate diagnosis, and biopsy of the bronchus may reveal other abnormalities such as a granuloma or a necrotizing vasculitis, for instance, Wegener's granulomatosis. Smears of secretions from areas of pathology may reveal organisms not evident in expectorated sputum, as in tuberculosis, and with proper technique one can obtain cultures from pneumonic lesions to evaluate the type of infection that is present. In addition, brushing of the surface of the airways followed by cytological study may reveal malignant cells, as well as fungi or other infecting agents. Finally, it is possible to obtain a sample of lung tissue directly through the bronchoscope in order to establish the nature of diffuse interstitial lung disease.

Although transbronchial biopsy is not infrequently associated with some degree of hemoptysis or with pneumothorax, neither of these complications is serious and the mortality is extremely low. This technique is the first approach to the patient with a visible solitary lesion on the x-ray film of the chest, presumably a carcinoma, or to the patient in whom physical or radiographic study suggests an obstructing lesion in the airways; to the patient with hemoptysis in whom the site must be identified and, if possible, the cause ascertained; and to the patient with diffuse lung disease that can only rarely be diagnosed with certainty by other techniques. In addition, the nature of a primary tumor may be revealed by transbronchial biopsy in a patient with what appears to be metastatic lesions to the lung, and the rare form of nodular sarcoid, which can mimic this appearance, can be excluded. Bronchoscopy may also be an important means of relieving airway obstruction either from a foreign body or from impacted secretions in a patient with atelectasis, and some have used the bronchofiberscope to provide lavage to the airways in patients with obstructive lung disease in respiratory failure. Finally, in patients with malignant cells in the sputum, bronchoscopic inspection and washing of lung segments may reveal a tumor not yet visible on the x-ray film of the chest.

Lung Aspiration and Biopsy

In some patients with pneumonia in whom it is not possible to induce the production of sputum or to obtain an adequate specimen by transtracheal aspiration, it may be advisable to aspirate material via a thin-walled needle directly from the area of pathology. Such aspiration of the lung has been associated with surprisingly few complications and is a way of insuring the appropriate antibiotic therapy, particularly in the immunocompromised host. Using fluoroscopic intensification, it is also possible, in skilled hands, to aspirate material from small peripheral lung nodules, not accessible to the bronchofiberscope, and, by cytological staining to make a diagnosis of lung cancer, even of the cell type. Needle biopsy of the lung, which involves a larger, cutting needle, is a means of obtaining pulmonary tissue, either from isolated lesions or from areas of diffuse lung disease, but this procedure is associated with risk of hemorrhage and of pneumothorax. It is probably not advisable to perform a cutting needle biopsy of a lung nodule because of the possibility of dissemination of tumor cells along the biopsy track if the lesion is malignant, a complication not associated with needle aspiration. The risk in patients with diffuse lung disease is probably too great to warrant performance of a procedure that yields such a limited amount of tissue as to be nondiagnostic often. When the diagnosis cannot be made by fiberoptic bronchoscopy in patients with diffuse lung disease, an open-lung biopsy is probably the procedure of choice.

Additional Reading

Bates DV, Macklem PT, Christie RV: Respiratory Function in Disease. Second edition. Philadelphia, W. B. Saunders, 1971.

Burrows B, Knudson RJ, Lebowitz MD: The relationship of childhood respiratory illness to adult obstructive airways disease. Am Rev Respir Dis 115:751, 1977.

Campbell EJM: Physical signs of diffuse airways obstruction and lung distension. Thorax 24:1–4, 1969.

Engel GL: A life setting conducive to illness: The giving-up–given up-complex. Ann Int Med 69:293, 1968.

Fishman AP: Pulmonary Diseases and Disorders. Vols. 1 and 2. New York, McGraw-Hill Book Co., 1981.

Forgacs P: The functional basis of pulmonary sounds. Chest 73:339–405, 1978.

Fraser, RG, Paré JAP: Diagnosis of Diseases of the Chest. Philadelphia, W. B. Saunders, 1970.

Guenter CA, Welch MH: Pulmonary Medicine. Philadelphia, J. B. Lippincott, 1977.

Nath AR, Capel LH: Inspiratory crackles— early and late. Thorax 29:223–227, 1974.

Sackner MA: Bronchofiberscopy. Am Rev Respir Dis 111:62–88, 1975.

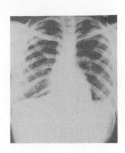

CHAPTER TWO

ASTHMA

Asthma is defined as reversible airways obstruction. It is characterized by hyperirritability of the airways. Substances that have no effect when inhaled by normal people cause bronchoconstriction in patients with asthma. The principal feature of the condition is extreme variability, both from patient to patient and from time to time in the same patient. It ranges from a mild wheeze with respiratory infection in children, which may disappear in later life, to severe, continuous, and even fatal obstruction of the airways. It may be present as a single entity, but some element of reversible bronchoconstriction frequently exists in patients with other types of chronic obstructive pulmonary disease. Asthma does not cause emphysema or other kinds of chronic disease, but itself may remain a significant cause of disability. It probably occurs at some time in the lives of between 5 and 10 per cent of the population. Because of its prevalence, because there is so much that the physician can do for patients with asthma, and because a great deal of interesting and important information has accumulated about the condition during recent years, an entire chapter of this book is devoted to it.

PATHOGENESIS

The principal pathogenetic feature of asthma is hyperirritability of the small and large airways within the lung. Even when normal, patients with asthma develop bronchoconstriction upon the inhalation of a wide variety of substances, such as very dilute concentrations of histamine, which have no effect on normal subjects. The tendency to bronchoconstriction is related to the autonomic nervous system. Although airway smooth muscle is not directly innervated by the sympathetic nervous system, it is rich in adrenergic receptors responsive to catecholamines liberated in the lung and elsewhere. In addition, the smooth muscle is directly innervated by the cholinergic system, which causes bronchoconstriction. The balance between adrenergic and cholinergic activity determines smooth muscle tone. There is some evidence that patients with asthma have relative blockade of the beta-adrenergic system, leaving unopposed the normal constricting action of the cholinergic system. This evidence is equivocal, and the beta-blockade

23

theory of asthma seems very implausible because of the fact that beta-blockade, which may be harmful and should be used with great caution in patients with asthma, does not cause asthma in normal subjects.

A more likely cause of the hyperirritable airways is overactivity of the parasympathetic system. Cholinergic nerve endings lying within the airways, known as irritant receptors, respond to the presence of various substances by causing, via a reflex arc up and down the vagus nerve, bronchoconstriction. It is not known whether or not there is a genetic tendency to hyperirritability of this system, but the well-known familial aggregation of asthma suggests that this may be the case. In addition, however, it is now known that a variety of agents, principally viral infections or even immunization with influenza vaccine, lead to transient hyperirritability of the airways in normal subjects. In all likelihood, such events have an effect on the irritant receptors, making them more sensitive to bronchoconstricting agents. This is why nonbacterial respiratory infection is such an important cause of worsening asthma in patients. Stimulation of the irritant receptors is probably responsible for the very common and most important symptom of asthma, the sensation of chest tightness, which may be independent of the actual constriction of airways.

Asthma has long been considered an allergic disease. It is certainly true that many patients with the condition have other forms of allergy and they come from allergic families. In addition, it is quite clear that in some patients, particularly children, allergic reactions may lead to bronchoconstriction. Many of the details of the mechanism of the allergic reaction have become apparent in recent years. Allergy to inhaled or even ingested antigen

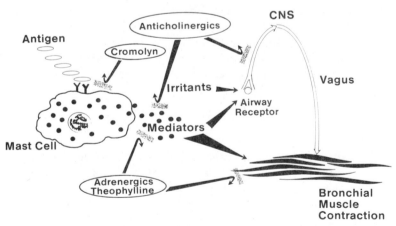

Figure 2–1 *Pathogenesis of asthma.* Inhaled or ingested antigen bridges IgE antibodies, coating the surface of mast cells, perhaps within the airway lumen, to cause mediator release. Cromolyn prevents this reaction by stabilizing the membrane of the mast cell. Stimulation of intracellular c-AMP by adrenergic drugs, and indirectly by theophylline, inhibits the release of mediators. These drugs also act directly on smooth muscle in the airways to reduce bronchoconstriction. The mediators released from mast cells, notably histamine, produce bronchoconstriction and also stimulate irritant receptors, which also respond directly to a variety of inhaled agents and local phenomena, such as the heat exchange induced by exercise, to cause reflex bronchoconstriction via the cholinergic arc. This is blocked by anticholinergic drugs, which also inhibit mediator release from mast cells.

is associated with increased concentrations of IgE antibodies in the blood and these antibodies become fixed on mast cells in the lung. Antigen then attaches to the surface of the mast cell, bridging these antibodies and leading to a series of reactions within the cell that result in the release of the many known mediators of asthma. These include histamine, slow-reacting substance of anaphylaxis, eosinophilic chemotactic factor, and a variety of other materials. It is interesting that many of the drugs that are used in the treatment of asthma have a major effect on this reaction. Mediator release is inhibited by increased concentrations of cyclic AMP within the mast cell and stimulated by increased concentrations of cyclic GMP. Beta-adrenergic drugs tend to increase the cyclic AMP, whereas cholinergic drugs increase cyclic GMP, so that the beneficial effects of beta-adrenergics in part stem from inhibition of mediator release from the sensitized mast cell. The enhancement of asthma induced by cholinergic stimulation may in part relate to increased release of mediators. In addition, cyclic AMP is broken down by phosphodiesterase, which is inhibited by theophylline, and this may be a major mechanism whereby theophylline is effective in the treatment of asthma.

The reactions that occur in the mast cell are similar to the reactions that occur in the smooth muscle, the final effector of bronchial constriction. Thus the action of the drugs is a dual one: indirect effects on smooth muscle via mediator release and direct bronchoconstriction and bronchodilation. It is now apparent that histamine, long thought to be an important cause of bronchoconstriction in allergic asthma, acts at least in part by stimulating the irritant receptors through the cholinergic reflex pathway mentioned previously. The interrelationships between the allergic reaction and reflex bronchoconstriction are complex. One of the puzzles in the past has been the fact that antigens, generally of large size and unable to cross the epithelial barrier of the airways, can provoke the allergic reaction. It now appears that the antigen reacts with mast cells lying on the surface of the airways, with subsequent mediator release and, possibly, increased permeability of the mucosa.

Although the reflex and the allergic mechanisms have been well worked out, other aspects of the airway obstruction are not so clear. These are the characteristic edema and inflammatory changes in the mucosa of the airways and the tenacious mucus plugs that are responsible for the most severe cases of asthma. Whether or not these changes are simply a consequence of the type of reaction described previously or whether they represent results of other unknown pathways is not clear. It is likely that the mucosal changes are the component of asthma that responds to steroid therapy, principally in view of the fact that steroids act slowly over a period of hours or days and do not appear to act by causing relaxation of smooth muscle. Mucus plugging is even less well understood. It may occur without other evidence of severe asthma, leading, occasionally, to atelectasis even in the absence of generalized wheeze. Experimentally, it has been shown to occur extremely quickly after allergic challenge to sensitive dogs. It is not known whether or not the mucus is abnormal in character, whether there is excessive formation of mucus, or whether there is impaired clearance. Whatever the cause, mucus plugging is the hallmark of fatal asthma, and although no effective therapy has been devised for this aspect of the condition, it should be borne in mind as being present in patients with severe symptoms.

CLINICAL FEATURES

The clinical features of asthma all stem from the airway obstruction. The principal, almost constant symptom of chest tightness may signal increased activity of irritant receptors or may be the result of bronchoconstriction. The one or more musical wheezes characteristic of asthma result from the turbulent flow of air through constricted airways. Dyspnea is clearly the result of the marked increased difficulty with breathing.

Evaluation of Severity

The severity of asthma is best reflected in some measurement of airway obstruction, most simply a measurement of peak expiratory flow rate (PEFR). Peak flow meters are very inexpensive; they can even be purchased by patients for following the course of their own illness and dictating therapy, as will be described later. This or another relevant measurement should always be made to obtain an accurate index of the severity of obstruction.

There are many other indices of airway obstruction. Spirometry reveals decreased flow rates throughout the vital capacity and, generally, a nearly parallel reduction of the vital capacity. Partially occluded airways tend to close completely during forced expiration, leading to increased residual volume and reduction of vital capacity. Patients with asthma have an increase in lung volume, reflected in an increased posteroanterior diameter

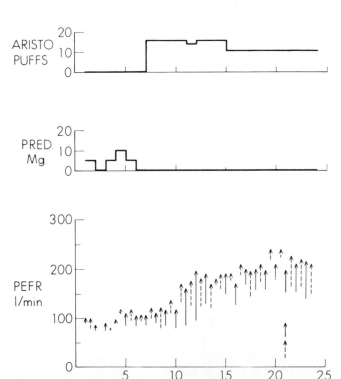

Figure 2–2 Value of measuring PEFR in a patient with asthma. Measurements were obtained by the patient before and after inhalation of isoproterenol in the morning (solid arrow) and in the afternoon (interrupted arrow). There is diurnal variation, PEFR usually being lower in the morning. PEFR remained low on 5 to 10 mg prednisone, improved promptly after starting treatment with triamcinolone acetonide aerosol (Aristocort), and remained elevated after prednisone was stopped and the dose of aerosol reduced from 16 to 12 puffs per day.

AIRWAY OBSTRUCTION

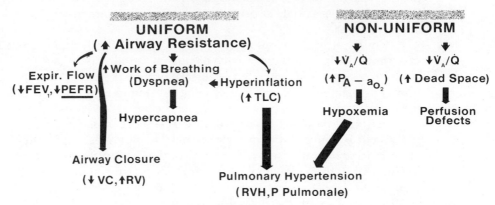

Figure 2–3 *Pathophysiology of asthma.* Uniform narrowing of airways causes the reduced expiratory flow rates characteristic of asthma. It also causes airway closure before the completion of expiration, leading to reduction of vital capacity (VC) and increase of residual volume (RV), and hyperinflation of the lung so as to overcome the resistance to breathing by increasing lung recoil. The increased airway resistance and hyperinflation increase the work of breathing, which is reflected in dyspnea. If this becomes overwhelming, the patient is unable to maintain an adequate alveolar ventilation and hypercapnia results.

Nonuniform obstruction to the airways causes abnormality of ventilation/perfusion (V̇/Q̇) ratios in different parts of the lung. Units in which the perfusion exceeds ventilation cause the hypoxemia characteristic of asthma. Underperfused units, often the result of local hyperinflation, cause an increase of physiological dead space and, hence, of ventilatory requirements. They may be evident as perfusion defects on lung scan and can be misinterpreted as pulmonary emboli. The hypoxemia, coupled with the hyperinflation of the lungs, causes pulmonary hypertension, which is reflected in electrocardiographic evidences of right ventricular hypertrophy.

of the chest, hyperlucency of the lungs, and an increased retrosternal air space on x-ray. This results from the fact that expiratory closure of the airway requires maintenance of high lung volume in order to permit expiration. There are two reasons for this. Airway diameter is increased at higher lung volumes because the increased recoil pressure of the distended lung, reflected in a more negative pleural pressure, pulls the airway open. In addition, the increased recoil pressure is translated into a higher alveolar pressure as the lung tends to deflate during expiration. In fact, the alveolar pressure is the effective driving pressure for expiration. Additional pressure generated by increasing pleural pressure through expiratory effort tends to compress the airways in addition to increasing alveolar pressure. This pressure is largely wasted, and the effective driving pressure for expiration becomes the elastic recoil pressure of the lung. In order to increase elastic recoil by inflating the lungs, patients with asthma tend to breathe at very high lung volumes, often near the total lung capacity. This provides maximal driving pressure for expiration, but the extra effort generated to maintain these volumes is a major component of the dyspnea.

Other manifestations of the disease are a reflection of the basic pathophysiology. In most cases, hyperventilation is a prominent feature because of attendant anxiety and stimulation of irritant receptors, and because incomplete emptying and filling of the lung lead to reflex stimulation to respiration. It is worth emphasizing at this point that when a patient with asthma fails to reveal hyperventilation or when the arterial P_{CO_2} is elevated, the asthma is very severe, and continuous and careful monitoring and treatment are essential. Patients with hypercapnia are at risk of dying from severe asthma.

A number of guidelines have been proposed for evaluating the severity of asthma, including the presence of pulsus paradoxus. It is known that the large pressure swing generated within the thorax because of airway obstruction is associated with inspiratory fall of systemic blood pressure, and there is a rough correlation between the degree of paradox and the severity of obstruction. Likewise, tensing of the accessory muscles of respiration is present in patients with severe obstruction. But these and other signs are often inaccurate and insensitive. They may be absent in patients with severe asthma, and their presence does not necessarily signify severe disease. Evaluation is best accomplished by an objective measurement of the airway obstruction, as with the peak flow meter.

Causes of Worsening

There are a great many known causes of asthma or, more correctly, causes of worsening obstruction, since it is rare that a single agent causes symptoms at any one time. Exacerbation of asthma usually results from a combination of factors superimposed upon the basic inherited or acquired hyperirritability of airways that is characteristic of the condition. Inhalation of antigens can cause bronchoconstriction in sensitive subjects, and the mechanism of this has been outlined. Particularly among children, sensitivity to house dust, pets, or other common environmental antigens may be important, but this is probably not the case for most adults. In the latter, nonbacterial respiratory infection is unquestionably the most important cause of worsening symp-

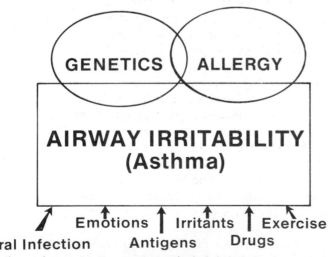

Figure 2–4 The fundamental characteristic of asthma is increased irritability of the airways. In many instances this appears to be related to the allergic state, and both atopy and airway irritability may have a genetic component. Airway irritability is increased by a wide variety of phenomena. Nonbacterial respiratory infections seem to be the most important cause of severe asthma. Suggestion is known to be associated with bronchoconstriction and bronchodilation, and emotional factors are undoubtedly important in many patients. In allergic subjects, inhaled or ingested antigens may provoke bronchoconstriction and a great many agents, particularly in industry, may cause bronchoconstriction either because of an allergic reaction or by a direct effect, as is the case with simple chemicals and pollutants such as ozone. Drugs, notably aspirin, cause bronchoconstriction because of their effect on prostaglandin metabolism and exercise produces bronchoconstriction in direct proportion to the amount of heat exchange in the airways.

toms. There is now a great deal of evidence indicating that viral and, possibly, mycoplasmic infections are associated with bronchoconstriction in patients with asthma. In contrast, there is no such association with bacterial infections, and there is no evidence that antibiotic therapy is of any benefit for the treatment of asthma. This is such as important relationship that when a patient with asthma develops pneumonia, if the asthma is not worse, it is most likely a bacterial infection; whereas if there is an exacerbation of asthma, one can be confident that a nonbacterial infection is present. A wide variety of chemicals have been identified as causing asthma in sensitive subjects, and a careful history of industrial exposure is very important. To what extent these agents act through a reflex or an allergic mechanism is incompletely understood.

Most physicians are convinced that emotional factors are extremely important, and various psychoanalytic formulations of asthma have been advanced. Although there is no clear evidence about this, there are certainly many patients who remain terribly sick with asthma despite maximum therapy and who become well when their personal situation and state of mind improve. Lack of self-respect, loneliness, grief, and guilt are among the feelings associated with worsening of asthma, and every effort should be made to improve the life situation. In addition, it is known that many patients with asthma are extremely susceptible to suggestion. Experiments have been performed in which patients with asthma were told they were being given bronchodilating drugs when they were actually being given bronchoconstricting agents, yet their measured airway resistance improved, indicating the powerful effect of the mind on overcoming even potent pharmacological agents. It is for this reason that so many useless therapies have flourished in the past and any new treatment for asthma must be based on careful, double-blind study. It is also for this reason that the pharmacological action of the potent drugs available for the treatment of asthma can and should be enhanced by the positive attitude of the physician. When separated from their parents, children with severe asthma often undergo remission, and patients under the personal supervision of a physician available to them generally do better than those who rely on episodic visits to emergency room and clinic. Clearly, the available and interested support of the physician plays an important role in the therapy of the disease.

Many other events lead to a worsening of asthma. A change of weather is frequently reported by patients as producing severe symptoms; and in our own hospital, the month of October, when it swings from warm to cool weather, is associated with the highest incidence of emergency room visits and admissions. Exercise is now known to produce bronchoconstriction in almost all patients with asthma, apparently because of heat loss from the respiratory tract induced by hyperventilation. One way to observe the induction of asthma in an asymptomatic subject is to measure expiratory flow rates before and after exercise.

There are a number of drugs, notably aspirin, that induce asthma in sensitive subjects, not by an allergic mechanism but, probably, by inhibition of the synthesis of bronchodilating prostaglandins. Aspirin sensitivity, generally associated with nasal polyps, is the prototype of this; but a number of other drugs act in the same fashion, including indomethacin and tartrazine yellow, widely used as a coloring agent in foods and in a variety of medications. Drug sensitivity is of sufficient importance that it is probably wise for an adult with asthma to avoid aspirin entirely, and in the puzzling case investigation of this type of reaction may reveal important leads.

Although, as discussed before, beta-blockade is not a convincing explanation for the hyperirritability of the airways that characterizes asthma, the beta-blocking agents that have no effect on normal airways can provoke intense bronchoconstriction in patients with asthma. This need not occur when the drug is first given but may slowly develop over a period of time, so that if such agents are needed for treatment of hypertension or cardiac arrhythmias, they must be given very cautiously, preferably by monitoring of peak expiratory flow rate. Even the beta-blocking eye drops timolol, used for the treatment of glaucoma, are absorbed in sufficient concentration to provoke worsening asthma in some patients.

Obviously the course of asthma is extremely variable. Most children who develop the condition improve as they approach puberty, many of them to be free of symptoms for the rest of their lives. When the disease develops in the adult, and it may appear for the first time at any age up to and including the eighties, it is more apt to be severe and less responsive to therapy. When asthma first develops, it is usually relatively mild and responsive to treatment, but as symptoms persist, if they do, the response to therapy becomes less complete. For this reason, although the mechanism of loss of responsiveness to therapy is not understood, it is wise only to give as much treatment as needed and when remission occurs to withdraw therapy promptly. Patients who develop asthma rarely become sick enough to enter the hospital during the first year of the illness, but thereafter severe asthma can occur at any time. In many instances, a very severe attack occurs only once or twice in a lifetime, though there are some patients who experience severe symptoms over and over again.

Diagnosis

A diagnosis of asthma is usually obvious from the history and examination. In patients who are asymptomatic at the time of evaluation, there may be difficulty, but one should carefully learn about the details of the symptoms, particularly asking abut the sensation of chest tightness, which is almost always present and relatively specific. If peak expiratory flow rate is normal, the patient can be asked to exercise; a decrease by 20 per cent or more is strongly suggestive of asthma. The patient can be given a peak flow meter to record measurements during times of health and respiratory distress and, then, after inhalation of a bronchodilating drug.

In patients with evident obstructive disease, musical wheezing is suggestive of asthma, but the diagnosis depends upon demonstration of reversibility. It must be emphasized that, in some patients, presumably those with severe mucus plugging, inhalation of a bronchodilator may have little effect, so that the measurements must be repeated many times before one can be sure that reversibility is not present. Changing values of peak expiratory flow rate from time to time are just as important as the acute change induced by inhalation of a bronchodilator. There are rare patients with seemingly irreversible pulmonary disease who respond dramatically to corticosteroid therapy, and they are probably individuals with asthma. Such patients generally have clumps of eosinophils in their sputum. A therapeutic trial of corticosteroids is warranted in such patients, but it must be coupled with measurements of expiratory flow rate so that the response can be documented. One must not rely on symptomatic improvement, which can be quite nonspecific with steroid therapy.

Differential Diagnosis

Acute asthma may be confused with pulmonary edema and pulmonary embolism. *Pulmonary edema* may be associated with wheezing (cardiac asthma), but the history and cardiac and radiographic findings should make the diagnosis clear. Patients with severe asthma are frequently hypertensive, which is not a contraindication to the use of adrenergic drugs; but pulmonary edema secondary to hypertension should be reflected in cardiomegaly, basilar crackles, and a history of progressive illness rather than episodic attacks of dyspnea. Chest tightness may be a useful clue in this situation. Pulmonary embolism has been mistakenly diagnosed in patients with asthma because of the belief that pulmonary embolism is associated with wheezing. This may be the case, but patients without obstructive lung disease who develop pulmonary embolism rarely have sufficient bronchoconstriction to produce wheezing. Thus, dyspnea associated with evident airway obstruction is almost certainly not the result of pulmonary embolism alone. It is important to note that patients with asthma often have perfusion defects on lung scan. This is probably due to the fact that some alveoli distal to partially obstructed bronchi became greatly overinflated. As a result the capillaries within their walls become so stretched and attenuated that they obstruct the circulation. These perfusion defects can be, and have been, misinterpreted as pulmonary emboli.

Upper airway obstruction can mimic asthma. Tracheal stenosis is a complication of intubation, which may have been performed for severe asthma. Patients with this condition have noisy respirations, but the stridor is generally a single note, dominant over the trachea and not associated with the musical wheezing of asthma. The patient will report that, even though dyspnea is present, there is no chest tightness and the distress is different from that associated with asthma. If there is any doubt, the physician can measure inspiratory flow rates as well as expiratory flow rates. Fixed obstruction of the upper airways is associated with just as much reduction of flow rate during inspiration as during expiration, whereas all types of obstructive lung disease lead to severe expiratory obstruction with relative preservation of inspiratory flow rates.

TREATMENT

General Principles

The treatment of asthma begins with the history. Any agents known to precipitate symptoms should be avoided. In addition to antigens, these particularly include the chemicals often found in industry, and drugs, especially aspirin. Mention has already been made of the importance of emotional factors, with emphasis on the importance of a positive attitude on the part of the physician; such an attitude enables the physician to utilize the beneficial effects of suggestion in treating the disease. The available, interested physician is clearly an effective force. It may be possible to suggest changes in living conditions, such as a return to work so as to develop self-respect and pride, or a change in occupation or even living conditions so as to have a more positive, joyous attitude towards life. Since viral infections are important causes of asthma, immunization with the appropriate influenza vaccine or other antiviral agents as they become available should be employed.

Allergy

Antiallergic therapy continues to be emphasized by many physicians, and although apparently of value in some children, it is of very limited value in adults. Clearly one should avoid exposure to animals, which is associated with bronchoconstriction, and the substitution of foam rubber for feather mattresses and pillows may be worthwhile. With limited exceptions, most notably asthma provoked by cat dander, injection therapy has not proven to be of value for the control of asthma, although it has been shown to be useful in patients with hay fever.

In recent years, cromolyn has been introduced as a specific agent for the treatment of allergic asthma. This drug, inhaled into the lung as a powder from a spinhaler (generally the contents of one capsule four times a day), is known to stabilize the membranes of the mast cell, preventing release of mediators when the sensitized cell is challenged with antigen. Most double-blind trials have revealed that cromolyn is effective in the treatment of asthma, with reduction of symptoms, and in children there seems to be some steroid-sparing effect. In adults, however, the benefit is less pronounced, and most older patients who have received cromolyn, even with initial benefit, find that the improvement is only moderate and does not permit reducing the dose of corticosteroids. Furthermore, the benefit is not lasting, and most patients discontinue the drug and find that their symptoms do not become worse. Nevertheless, there are indications for the use of this agent in the treatment of asthma. In individuals known to be sensitive to antigen who cannot avoid exposure the agent may be used prophylactically with profit. It also has some effect on preventing the asthma that follows exercise and may be used in the same fashion by athletes or by others who merely wish to exercise for pleasure. Finally, in adults with continuing symptoms a trial of cromolyn therapy is probably worthwhile. It must be emphasized that cromolyn is neither a bronchodilator nor an anti-inflammatory agent, and patients must understand that they use the drug to prevent the symptoms of asthma, not to control them. There are no serious side effects from the drug, although in some individuals it is irritating and may even provoke bronchoconstriction. For this reason, and in order to maximize delivery to the airways, its use may be preceded by an inhalation of isoproterenol.

Drugs

The major drugs used for the treatment of asthma are bronchodilators and corticosteroids. The most important principle of therapy is to use as much medication as needed to control symptoms or, preferably, to maintain maximum PEFR, but to use no more medication than is necessary. It is important to treat developing obstruction in the early stages in order to prevent severe obstruction with mucus plugging. Patients must learn how to use medication properly, to start treatment promptly as symptoms first appear, to maintain regular dosage schedules, and to reduce the dose of medication (when they get well) gradually rather than abruptly so as to avoid a sudden exacerbation of symptoms. It is desirable for patients to know as much as possible about their medications so that, with the help of their physician, they can constantly evaluate and revise their dosage requirements. In some instances, treatment can be started before symptoms develop, as with patients who know they will develop an exacerbation of asthma with a viral respiratory infection. Prophylaxis is much easier than treatment after airway obstruction has developed.

Bronchodilators

The principal bronchodilators are beta-adrenergic agents and theophylline. They both act by increasing the concentration of cyclic AMP in smooth muscle, which is associated with bronchodilation. In addition, they inhibit the release the mediators of asthma from mast cells by the same mechanism. When given by mouth, they probably act synergistically because neither can be given in a maximally effective dosage because of side effects.

Isoproterenol   It is quite clear that administration of *adrenergic drugs* by

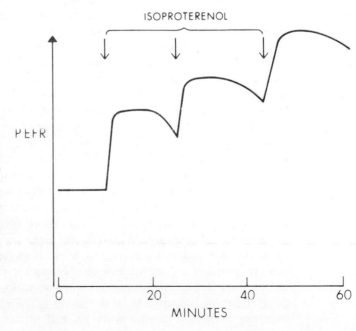

Figure 2-5 Three sequential inhalations of isoproterenol (↓) demonstrating the immediate onset of action on peak expiratory flow rate (PEFR); it peaks within 2 minutes but then declines in about 10 minutes. The second and third inhalations produce even more effect than the initial treatment because of better penetration of the aerosol into previously obstructed airways.

aerosol makes it possible to produce maximal bronchodilation with very, very small doses, in contrast to the limited effect on the airways produced by oral agents. Until recent years isoproterenol was the principal adrenergic aerosol available for treatment of asthma. It is now known that far less than the amount of isoproterenol contained in one puff in the available freon nebulizers, approximately 0.08 mg, produces a full effect on expiratory flow rates. It is also known that full bronchodilation is only achieved by successive inhalations of the drug 2 to 5 times every 20 minutes after the initial dose. This is because the bronchodilation produced by the initial dose leads to better distribution of subsequent doses through previously obstructed airways. Because isoproterenol has a half-life of about 7 minutes, it is not surprising that its maximal effect lasts no more than 10 minutes and then declines rapidly. For maximally effective therapy, the drug must be given every 20 minutes until a full effect is achieved. In some patients, continuing inhalation is necessary at similar intervals in order to maintain the effect. In others, once the airways are dilated they do not constrict again, at least for some time.

Patients must be given careful instruction in the use of aerosols. They must learn to inhale the drug into their lungs by actuating the nebulizer at the beginning of inspiration rather than at the end. It is not known whether the best effect is achieved by inhaling the agent after a maximal or normal expiration, but probably there is little difference between the two types of inhalation. The important point is to teach the patient to inhale the drug into the lungs, and the physician must watch the patient inhale the aerosol to make sure that the technique is correct.

Many physicians and patients are concerned about dangers of isoproterenol, but these have been greatly over-rated. Reports of paradoxical bronchoconstriction following inhalation of a bronchodilator have been poorly controlled and can be explained by the marked variability of asthma and by the known effects of suggestion. There is now considerable evidence that significant tolerance does not develop to the beta-adrenergic agents and that continuing use, even for many years, is not followed by substantial loss of effect. In addition, it has been shown that, in patients with asthma, inhalation of up to 5 puffs every 20 minutes is without effect on heart rate and rhythm. As long as the airways are obstructed and flow through them is turbulent, drug is deposited primarily in them and does not reach the alveoli for systemic absorption. Because of the short half-life, cumulative effects cannot occur if the inhalation is no more frequent than every 20 minutes. Thus, it appears quite safe to use this drug, one puff at a time, every 20 minutes, as needed.

Much of the concern about isoproterenol is related to the association between excessive deaths from asthma in the United Kingdom in the 1960's and the concurrent increasing sales of a concentrated form of the drug. This association probably was more coincidence than anything else, since other countries in which there were increasing sales of concentrated drug did not report increasing deaths. Many of the excessive deaths were among patients who did not use isoproterenol at all, and in almost all instances of fatal asthma that were examined pathologically there was overwhelming obstruction of the airways with mucus plugs. It is more likely that the increased deaths were related to the fact that in the early 1960's patients became somewhat casual about the care of their asthma; they no longer had available to them private physicians who came to the home and provided treatment until they either were well or were hospitalized. Following the publicity about deaths from asthma, patients became more concerned and sought treatment when their symptoms became severe, and the death rate declined. It is certainly true that when asthma becomes severe, aerosol may be totally ineffective because of imperfect penetration through plugged airways. Under these circumstances intensive therapy with systemic medication is mandatory. Refractoriness to isoproterenol represents inadequate penetration of the drug, not lack of pharmacological effect. It has been shown that patients who appear to be refractory still respond to injection of an adrenergic agent, and as soon as the obstruction improves they again respond to aerosol. Thus, patients must be informed about the dangers of worsening asthma, particularly if refractory to isoproterenol therapy, and the need to seek medical attention.

Metaproterenol, Terbutaline, and Salbutamol A number of new beta-adrenergic agents have been developed in the belief that they would provide selective action on the beta$_2$ receptors in the airways and not on the cardiovascular beta$_1$ receptors. Since aerosol isoproterenol can be given with safety and full effect without significant cardiovascular reaction, the need for these agents for aerosol treatment of asthma is less. However, these new drugs, which include metaproterenol, terbutaline, and salbutamol, have the additional advantage of a much longer duration of action. It has been shown that these agents produce almost as prompt and just as potent an effect on the airways as isoproterenol and that instead of lasting 20 to 30 minutes they last for 3 to 6 hours. Thus, in many patients who get good relief from isoproterenol but complain about having to use the drug frequently, substitution of metaproterenol, the new beta$_2$ stimulant available in this country as an aerosol, is often very successful. However, other patients claim that they do

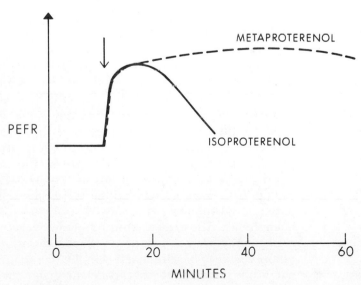

Figure 2-6 Comparison of a single dose of metaproterenol with isoproterenol aerosol. Both drugs produce a similar rapid effect on PEFR, but whereas the effect of isoproterenol begins to decline in about 10 minutes and is gone within the hour, metaproterenol causes continuing improvement for over an hour and remains in full effect for several hours.

not get as immediate or as pronounced an effect from this drug as they have experienced from isoproterenol, and they prefer to continue with the earlier drug. In order to achieve maximal effect, metaproterenol also must be inhaled sequentially, generally 1 puff every 10 minutes to a total of 3 doses.

The new beta-adrenergic drugs have an additional advantage of being active when taken by mouth. In the past, the only adrenergic agent available by mouth for the treatment of asthma was ephedrine. This drug acts by depleting catecholamine stores, and resistance soon develops. It has been shown with metaproterenol and with terbutaline, the oral agents available in this country, that minimal, if any, resistance develops. It is of interest that resistance to the major side effect, muscle tremor, does develop. Chronic tolerance studies have shown that although the airways remain just as responsive after institution of therapy, at least with regard to immediate effects of the drug, there is suppression of the action of the agent on the striated muscle receptors that are responsible for the tremor experienced by patients by jitteriness or nervousness. Thus, patients can be told when they start taking the drug that they may experience nervousness and jitteriness but that if they continue treatment these symptoms will subside within a few days. In some instances, they can cut the dose in half until sufficient tolerance develops to allow them to resume full dosage.

There is now evidence that oral agents add very little to the action of aerosol. Much more effect can be produced on flow rates by tiny doses of aerosol, which are without systemic effect, than can be produced by the oral agents. Clearly the most effective treatment of asthma is the regular use of an adrenergic aerosol. However, many patients prefer to take a pill, and continuing therapy is most practically carried out by the administration of metaproterenol or terbutaline every 6 to 8 hours. This can be supplemented by isoproterenol or metaproterenol aerosol for worsening symptoms. In addition, there is some evidence that agents reach receptors in small airways that are not reached by the aerosol, so that the combined routes of administration may have some advantage. We frequently give our patients 20 mg of metaproterenol or 5 mg of terbutaline every 6 to 8 hours and supplement this with isoproterenol as needed for symptoms or reduction of PEFR.

Theophylline The other principal bronchodilator is theophylline. This drug cannot be taken by aerosol because of its unpleasant taste. In recent years, it has been shown that the effectiveness of theophylline is clearly related to the concentration of the drug in the blood and that the higher the concentration the greater the effect. It has also been shown that toxicity increases with increasing blood levels. The current recommendation is that blood levels be maintained between 10 and 20 micrograms per milliliter, which is effective and free of side effects. The cheapest and simplest method of administration of theophylline is by aminophylline tablets, but in some patients the choline salt (choledyl) is better tolerated; others prefer liquid elixophyllin. The drug should be given every 6 to 8 hours at a dose of 0.5 mg/kg body weight per hour. Blood level should then be measured just before a dose to be sure that it is in the therapeutic range. If it is not, the dose should be increased. Most physicians give a theophylline preparation along with the adrenergic therapy described previously.

It is important to note that a number of factors affect theophylline metabolism and, hence, blood levels. Cigarette smoking increases the rate of theophylline degradation and smokers require more theophylline than nonsmokers to maintain an effective blood level. A patient who stops smoking may have to decrease the theophylline dose. A number of drugs inhibit theophylline metabolism, notably erythromycin; and if this antibiotic is given for a respiratory infection, it may be necessary to reduce the theophylline dose. Worsening or improvement of liver function is associated with reduction or increase of theophylline metabolism, respectively, requiring the appropriate change of dosage.

Theophylline is also available for intravenous use, to be described later for the treatment of severe asthma, and as rectal suspensions, which have been shown to produce very effective blood levels quite promptly. In some patients, whose asthma worsens in the night, rectal theophylline will provide sufficient blood levels to insure comfortable sleep.

Theophylline therapy is often limited by gastrointestinal intolerance, which probably results from action on the central nervous system and is related to the blood level of theophylline. But some patients, particularly if they are given intravenous therapy, develop much more serious central nervous system disturbances, starting with hyperirritability and nervousness and ending in convulsions, before the warning signs of gastrointestinal discomfort have appeared. It is for this reason that patients given large amounts of theophylline must be monitored with measurement of their blood level.

In recent years long-acting theophylline preparations have been developed, permitting maintenance of a much more constant blood level with only twice daily administration of the drug. These agents can be substituted, at the same total dosage, for the conventional preparations, but again blood levels should be checked to be sure that the dose is sufficient and safe. The advantage of this preparation is that the blood level can be measured at any time, whereas for the short-acting preparations the peak effect can only be gauged by measurement within 30 to 60 minutes of administration and the minimal level can only be assessed by making a measurement prior to the next dose. Thus the principal advantage of the long-acting preparations is a relatively constant blood level. The major disadvantage, in addition to expense, is that the disappearance time is much longer, so that if toxicity develops it will persist longer.

Anticholinergic Drugs   Also effective as bronchodilators are anticholinergic drugs, but they are limited by the fact that to produce bronchodilation they have to be given in toxic amounts. Atropine and the recently developed SCH 1000 have been given by aerosol with beneficial results, but the general experience has been that these agents produce no more bronchodilation than isoproterenol; they do not produce an additive effect to that drug, and in many patients the effect is less than that obtained with beta-adrenergics. This is somewhat surprising in view of the important contribution of cholinergic activity to bronchoconstriction. It is possible that the limited effectiveness of these drugs relates to imperfect deposition in the tracheobronchial tree and absorption into the airways; if an aerosol could be developed that was more topically active, it might have an important role in the treatment of asthma. Physicians have long been concerned that atropine might produce drying of secretions, as it does the mouth, but there is really no evidence to support this fear, and it is just as likely that reduction of secretions from the tracheobronchial tree would be helpful as it is that it would be harmful.

Corticosteroids   The most effective and, at the same time, the most toxic agents used for the treatment of asthma are corticosteroids. Their mechanism of action is not entirely clear. It is known that they do not inhibit the immediate Type 1 allergic reaction, do not act principally as bronchodilators, and develop their effect relatively slowly. It has been shown that administration of a single dose of steroids leads to beginning improvement of pulmonary function within two hours, reaching a maximum in eight hours. Continuing therapy leads to further improvement over three to five days. There is some evidence that corticosteroids enhance the bronchodilating action of adrenergic drugs, but this is contradictory. It is likely that the major effect of these drugs is on the inflammatory changes in the airways.

In the past, prednisone was given to patients with asthma when they failed to respond or remain well on maximum therapy with bronchodilating drugs. It can be given with the expectation that asthma will improve. The major principle of therapy has always been to give as much steroid as needed to induce improvement and, then, to taper the dose just as rapidly as possible. Patients must be cautioned not to taper too quickly, certainly not to discontinue the drug immediately, for fear of serious exacerbation of symptoms. Patients requiring continuous treatment with oral steroids may be switched to therapy on alternate days in order to preserve adrenal function, but in many such instances the symptoms of asthma are so severe on the day off therapy as to make this treatment unsatisfactory. It is generally felt that a maintenance dose of less than 10 mg per day is without significant toxicity, and there is evidence that such dosages are not associated with an increased risk of tuberculosis, peptic ulcer disease, hypertension, diabetes, or osteoporosis.

Most patients with asthma respond to initial treatment with steroids, but many individuals, particularly those on chronic therapy, seem to become less responsive with time. It is not clear whether or not resistance to the drug is induced by the continuing use of the agent or, rather, is simply due to increasingly refractory asthma. It is certainly wise to reduce the dose of steroids to a minimum, if possible to eliminate them entirely, and only to use them for acute exacerbations. It is in this area particularly that careful adherence to the prescription is important. It has been shown that patients who maintain careful records and take the drugs as prescribed actually require less steroid therapy and remain freer of symptoms than patients who take the drug intermittently and haphazardly. A typical schedule of steroid therapy would be the institution of 30 mg of prednisone a day in divided doses until the patient remains well, and then tapering the dose of the drug by 5 mg every three days as long as symptoms are absent. Recurrence of symptoms necessitates a higher dosage. It must be added, however, that this is extremely variable; the initial dose, the length of time it is needed, and the rate at which it can be tapered vary tremendously. All patients must learn for themselves how the drug should be used.

Beclomethasone dipropionate, available as Vanceril and Beclovent, is a steroid aerosol that exerts a topical action on the airways without producing the side effects associated with oral steroid therapy. This drug is administered from a freon nebulizer in a 50 mcg puff. It is generally given in a starting dose of 8 to 12 puffs per day. It is known that up to 1 mg of the drug, 20 puffs, is without any significant effect on adrenal function, and there is evidence that one puff of the drug is approximately equivalent to the administration of 1 mg of prednisone by mouth. It has been clearly shown in a large number of double-blind controlled trials that this drug is an effective agent for the treatment of asthma. Approximately 75 per cent of steroid-dependent asthmatics can discontinue the use of oral steroids and maintain full control or even improvement of their asthma. Particularly striking is the fact that steroid-dependent patients with overt evidence of hydrocorticism can maintain control of asthma when they switch to steroid aerosol, but the systemic evidence of the steroid effect disappears. This has represented the major difficulty with the substitution of aerosol for oral steroids since many patients develop arthralgias, myalgias, and, particularly, nasal stuffiness. These symptoms will disappear with time, but they are an indication of adrenal insufficiency. Nasal stuffiness is probably due to allergic rhinitis that has been unmasked by discontinuation of systemic corticosteroid. It often responds to topical therapy with dexamethasone (Decadron) spray. It is probably wise to continue daily doses of a short-acting steroid, such as 20 mg of hydrocortisone, until adrenal function has returned to normal. Ideally this would be measured by stimulation tests of adrenal function, but a practical approach in the patient who has been maintained on more than 10 mg of prednisone per day and is switched to steroid aerosol is to give the hydrocortisone for 9 to 12 months, which provides adequate replacement without preventing return of normal adrenal function.

As mentioned, about 75 per cent of steroid-dependent asthmatics can be well maintained on an aerosol. About one half of these require short bursts of oral steroid therapy for severe exacerbations of asthma, notably after a nonbacterial respiratory infection. Some patients learn to start taking prednisone as soon as they develop a viral infection and, then, quickly taper off the drug in three to five days. In about 25 per cent of patients the aerosol is less effective. Many of these are patients who remain symptomatic on high doses of oral steroids, and they probably represent truly steroid-resistant patients. In some of these individuals the aerosol is useful in reducing the steroid requirements, but there is a group of asthmatic patients who remain symptomatic despite full therapy with all drugs. As indicated earlier in this chapter many of these patients appear to suffer from severe emotional problems and improvement of asthma only follows their resolution. The only toxic effect ascribed to steroid aerosols is oral candidiasis, which has been reported in a variable number of patients. This responds quickly to an antifungal mouthwash or to reduction of the aerosol dose. It has not proven to be of serious consequence, and in one controlled study it was no more common in patients taking steroid aerosol than those taking placebo. It is certainly no contraindication to the use of these drugs.

The most important consideration in the use of steroid aerosols is the fact that if severe asthma develops, the patient must promptly start using oral steroids. As with isoproterenol, the development of severe obstruction prevents the aerosol from effectively reaching the sites in the airways where it is needed. Deaths have been reported, particularly in children, who were successfully switched to steroid aerosol but subsequently developed asthma and died because they did not realize that they needed oral steroids. All patients must be carefully instructed to keep oral steroids on hand and if asthma worsens to start taking them.

In some patients, the dominant manifestation of asthma is distressing cough, often at night and usually dry and irritating. The act of coughing is known to produce bronchoconstriction and may be associated with audible wheeze and increasing dyspnea. In these patients, 15 mg of codeine may be a useful adjunct to therapy.

SEVERE ASTHMA (STATUS ASTHMATICUS)

Severe asthma requires special attention and treatment. Although most commonly encountered in hospital emergency rooms today, it still may be a problem for physicians in the office or even in the home. Evaluation of severity and of response to treatment is best accomplished by measurement of PEFR, and one guideline is the presence of a PEFR of less than 100 L/min. If the peak flow remains low after initial therapy with an adrenergic agent and theophylline, the patient probably should be hospitalized immediately. Patients with severe asthma must also receive measurements of arterial blood gas composition, and if the Pco_2 is normal (40 mm Hg) or higher, they should also be hospitalized.

Treatment

Drugs

Treatment should be started immediately with an adrenergic agent, either the subcutaneous injection of 0.3 to 0.5 ml of epinephrine (1:1000 dilution), which can be given every 20 minutes, or of terbutaline, which has recently become available in the United States but has not yet been proven to be of greater efficacy than epinephrine. If the patient is known not to have been taking theophylline, an initial infusion of aminophylline, 6 mg per kg, can be given over a 20 minute period. One must be very careful that no theophylline has been taken at all during the past 24 hours, since patients on chronic theophylline therapy often have surprisingly high blood levels even though they deny recent use of the drug. If there is any question about previous use of theophylline, it is best simply to start maintenance therapy at the recommended rate of 0.5 mg per kg per hour in normal subjects and at half that rate in patients with congestive heart failure, liver disease, or significant hypoxemia. With continuing therapy the theophylline blood level should be determined and the dosage adjusted to provide the therapeutic range of from 10 to 20 mcg/ml. In patients who are to be hospitalized corticosteroids should also be started. It has been shown that, in untreated patients, an infusion containing 300 mg of hydrocortisone per day is as effective as much higher doses, but in patients who have been taking steroids it is probably better to give 1 to 1.5 gm of hydrocortisone per day in order to obtain a full effect. It is important to remember that steroids will not begin to have an effect for several hours and that one must rely on intensive therapy with other agents until their action becomes evident. As the obstruction improves, therapy can be reduced. In patients not previously taking steroids in whom improvement occurs very rapidly, corticosteroids can be discontinued entirely in 2 to 3 days. More often the condition improves slowly, and it is necessary to treat with oral steroids, starting with administration of the drug every eight hours in order to maintain the therapeutic effect around the clock. The patient can then be started on steroid aerosol and the oral drug tapered as rapidly as judged possible by maintenance of a satisfactory PEFR.

Monitoring

Patients hospitalized with severe asthma require continuous monitoring, both of expiratory flow rates and of heart rate and rhythm. They frequently need intravenous fluids because of dehydration, and hypovolemia has been shown to be a cause of hypotension in some dehydrated patients with asthma. Arterial blood gases must be measured initially. If the Pco_2 is reduced, as it is in most patients, the measurement need not be repeated unless there is deterioration of PEFR. Most patients will reveal some degree of hypoxemia, and it is wise to administer oxygen by nasal catheter or Venturi mask, but usually arterial unsaturation is mild and is not of great consequence to the patient. Mucus plugs are undoubtedly present in most or all patients with status asthmaticus. Although there is no satisfactory treatment for this potentially lethal component of asthma, chest clapping with encouragement of coughing is worth trying. If this results in expectoration of plugs, which can easily be seen by suspending the sputum in saline, it should be continued.

Under no circumstances should the patient hospitalized with asthma be given any sedatives or tranquilizers. It has been the experience in a number of centers that administration of these drugs to the patient seriously ill with asthma may be associated with sudden and unexpected death. This probably relates to the fact that the patient with severe airway obstruction requires maximal effort simply to maintain an adequate ventilation. If respiratory drive and conscious awareness of the severity of asthma is in any way blunted, respiration may be depressed, with ensuing apnea. Where these drugs have been banished for hospitalized patients, there has been a reduction in the number of sudden unexpected deaths from asthma. It is probably safe to administer tranquilizers to anxious outpatients, but even they must be cautioned not to use these drugs if asthma becomes severe. It is worth noting that 24-hour monitoring of hospitalized patients has revealed that airway obstruction is apt to be much greater at night than during the day. In fact, most instances of sudden worsening occur at night. The reason for this is not clear. It is not related to the circadian rhythm of endogenous steroid secretion, but it means that the hospitalized patient requires particularly careful attention at night.

Artificial Ventilation

Most patients hospitalized with severe asthma will improve promptly, generally over a period of several days, and even patients hospitalized with hypercapnia often reveal improvement and reduction of arterial Pco_2 to the expected low value within a short period of time. A few patients, however, remain refractory to therapy and require endotracheal intubation with artificial ventilation. Intubation is obviously necessary in the patient who presents with apnea from overwhelming airway obstruction, but the indications for the procedure in other patients are not quite so obvious. It should be borne in mind that artificial ventilation has no effect on the expiratory obstruction, which is the dominant feature of asthma and other types of obstructive lung disease. Just as increasing expiratory effort fails to increase expiratory flow rates, because of airway closure, so too negative pressure at the mouth would not improve expiratory flow rates. Both volume and pressure respirators are designed to inflate the lungs and are only of value to the extent that the patient fails to make maximal inspiratory efforts. Thus, an obtunded patient with neuromuscular weakness or fatigue requires artificial ventilation, but most patients with asthma are alert and frightened and are making maximal inspiratory efforts themselves, so that they cannot be helped by artificial ventilation. It is only when, in association with progressive hypercapnia, they become fatigued and fail to make maximal efforts that artificial ventilation is of value and indicated. This means that the severely obstructed patient requires very careful observation, that an endotracheal tube and laryngoscope must be at hand to provide intubation if worsening occurs, and this may happen extremely rapidly, but that there is no set value of Pco_2 or other laboratory parameter that dictates the need for this procedure. Intubation is followed by a significant incidence of tracheal complications, and it should only be performed if necessary as well as useful.

COMPLICATIONS

There is now clear evidence that asthma itself does not lead to permanent changes in the lungs. Specifically, emphysema is not associated with asthma of even long duration and severity. Asthma may remain chronic and severe, with continuing symptoms and disability, but this is not associated with alveolar destruction or with other structural changes in the lungs. This may be of some comfort to patients who frequently have been told that they now have emphysema, and the reassurance that this is not the case, best based on pulmonary function measurements, may be very important.

Cor Pulmonale

In some patients with chronic continuing airway obstruction and hypoxemia, cor pulmonale may develop with evidence of congestive heart failure. This is the result of the sustained hyperinflation of the lung, with resultant increase in pulmonary vascular resistance and secondary increase in right heart pressures. It is uncommon in uncomplicated asthma and when it occurs, as in obstructive lung disease in general, it can be treated with diuretics. But it is not an indication for the use of digitalis. Acute cor pulmonale, also the result of hyperinflation of the lung, is common in severe asthma and is generally associated with EKG changes. P pulmonale is present in up to 25 per cent of patients with acute asthma and disappears as the airway obstruction improves.

Atelectasis

In some patients, mucus plugging of the airways can lead to atelectasis with total collapse of a lobe or even of one lung. This may occur in the absence of generalized airway obstruction, suggesting that mucus plugging is a phenomenon of different pathogenesis than bronchoconstriction. When present, it may be associated with chest tightness and dyspnea, but it is generally self-limited and of little consequence. Bronchoscopy may be employed in an attempt to aspirate obstructing secretions, but usually the secretions are in such small airways that this is unsuccessful. Expansion of the lung is more apt to occur after chest clapping and induced coughing with, ultimately, expectoration of the characteristic mucus plugs. Obstruction of segmental or smaller bronchi may lead to smaller areas of atelectasis. These may appear on the x-ray film of the chest and represent a source of concern but are of little consequence. The diagnosis is usually evident when they clear, but a persistent density may require bronchoscopy in order to exclude other causes of obstruction.

Pneumothorax

Nonuniform obstruction of airways may also lead to overexpansion of some alveoli with alveolar rupture. If this occurs near the surface of the lung, the result is pneumothorax, and all patients with asthma with worsening dyspnea should have an x-ray film of the chest to exclude this possibility. Significant collapse of the lung is best treated with introduction of a chest tube.

Pneumomediastinum

In some patients, alveoli deep within the lung may rupture from their attachments along the peribronchial and perivascular sheaths, so that the air will not dissect into the pleural space but goes to the mediastinum and then into the neck. Pneumomediastinum is generally associated with chest discomfort, palpable crepitus in the neck, and visible lines on the PA films of the chest. This is a dramatic but benign complication of asthma. It may also occur in normal subjects, and it requires no treatment other than observation to be sure that the dissection does not rupture into the pleura with pneumothorax.

Bronchopulmonary Aspergillosis

Some patients with asthma develop colonization of their airways with aspergillus. Bronchopulmonary aspergillosis can be associated with a particularly intractable form of asthma. It is usually accompanied by eosinophilia and frequently by a central type of bronchiectasis. Diagnosis is confirmed by serologic tests. Treatment is not directed at the fungus infection, which is largely ineffectual, but at the asthma, and corticosteroids are often needed.

SPECIAL CLINICAL PROBLEMS

Pregnancy

Pregnancy may pose special problems for the patient with asthma. There is evidence that patients with mild asthma are apt to improve when they become pregnant, but patients with more severe asthma, particularly if the pregnancy is unwanted, may become worse. Every effort should be made to avoid therapy with systemic drugs, which may affect the fetus, and to rely on adrenergic and steroid aerosols. If these agents are inadequate, one may be forced to employ theophylline and oral steroids.

Other Disease

Other diseases do not pose problems for patients with asthma, except with regard to difficulties caused by drug interactions, particularly with corticosteroids. The potentially hazardous effects of beta-blockers in patients who also have hypertension or heart disease has already been discussed. The use of corticosteroids for the control of asthma may make the control of *diabetes* more difficult, but the substitution of steroid aerosols can prevent this problem. Asthma does not appear to be particularly common in patients with *tuberculosis*, but the risk of rapidly progressive disease in an undiagnosed patient makes the prophylactic use of isoniazid prudent in steroid-dependent patients who have a positive tuberculin test. On the other hand, there have been some reports suggesting that the risk of a patient with asthma developing tuberculosis is so slight as not to warrant such therapy. Chemotherapeutic agents are so effective in the treatment of active tuberculosis that there is no contraindication to the simultaneous use of corticosteroids if it is needed for the control of asthma.

Adrenal insufficiency should cause an increased requirement for corticosteroid therapy of asthma, and there have been reports of patients in whom asthma was the presenting symptom of Addison's disease.

Surgery

Surgery is rarely a special problem for patients with asthma, since the airway obstruction can be well controlled with medication. Asthma is not a contraindication to thoracic surgical procedures, but, as in all obstructive lung disease, evaluation for surgery must take into consideration the patient's pulmonary function. Anesthesia itself represents little hazard, and ether anesthesia has even been used for the treatment of severe asthma. Of course, patients with asthma who have been treated with corticosteroids must be given adequate replacement therapy for any stress, particularly an operative procedure, and steroid requirements for control of asthma may be increased in the patient who is anxious about an impending operation. On the other hand, I have seen more than one patient in whom asthma and pulmonary function actually improved after successful resection of carcinoma of the lung.

Drug Abuse

Asthma may be a very difficult problem in patients being treated for drug abuse, largely because it is so difficult to insure compliance in these unfortunate patients. A well-structured drug-treatment program, which implies regular visits for administration of methadone, can have a positive impact on the treatment of asthma, just as it has had on the treatment of tuberculosis, by insuring that the patient takes the indicated chemotherapy.

Additional Reading

Austen KF, Lichtenstein LM (eds): Asthma. New York, Academic Press, 1973.
McFadden SR Jr, Feldman NT: Asthma: pathophysiology and clinical bronchitis. Med Clin North Am 61(6)1229–1238, 1977.
Weiss EB (ed): Status Asthmaticus. Baltimore, University Park Press, 1978.
Weiss EB, Segal MS (eds): Bronchial Asthma. Boston, Little, Brown & Co., 1970.
Williams MH Jr, Shim C: Asthma: Discussion in Patient Management. New York, Medical Examination Publishing Company, 1976.

CHAPTER THREE

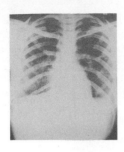

CHRONIC AIRWAY DISEASE AND EMPHYSEMA

A great many patients are victims of chronic airway obstruction, sometimes from asthma and sometimes from other conditions. Airway obstruction is usually due to abnormalities in the tracheobronchial tree, but it may result from emphysema. Some diseases of the airway may be associated with little obstruction to airflow. This chapter will be devoted to a description of specific entities — bronchitis, bronchiectasis and emphysema — and, then, the common clinical condition chronic obstructive pulmonary disease and its relationship to these disorders.

BRONCHITIS

Definition and Pathogenesis

Chronic bronchitis is defined as excessive secretion of mucus and is reflected in chronic cough productive of sputum. Pathologically it is characterized by enlargement of the mucus glands in the large airways, often without evidence of inflammatory changes. The latter are frequently present, however, in patients with associated bacterial infections. Bronchitis is largely due to the inhalation of cigarette smoke, which, presumably, has a directly irritant effect on the airways, but it is occasionally present in nonsmokers. Occupational pollution, particularly among miners, has been shown to be an important contributing cause, and there is evidence that people living in an urban environment have more bronchitis than those who live in the country. The condition is important in large part because of complications and associated disease, particularly chronic obstructive pulmonary disease (COPD). Bronchitis is frequently associated with narrowing and inflammatory changes of the small airways, termed bronchiolitis, which is probably also due to cigarette smoking and which is probably the major cause of COPD (see page 56). Thus, chronic cough alerts the physician to the presence of bronchitis in a smoker and to the likelihood that small airways disease is also present, which may lead to significant trouble, if it is not present already.

Clinical Evaluation

The principal concern in the patient with chronic bronchitis must be the development of obstructive airways disease. For this reason, all patients should receive spirometry. The presence of airway obstruction, or its development during followup examination, which should always include annual spirometry in smokers, indicates increased urgency to discontinue cigarette smoking. It has been clearly shown in large studies that the FEV_1 deteriorates more rapidly, albeit slowly, over the years in smokers with chronic bronchitis than in nonsmokers and that this accelerated decline reverts to the normal, very slow deterioration if smoking is stopped. It has also been shown that the chronic cough, also associated with smoking, is not clearly correlated with severity of obstructive disease and the two phenomena, mucus gland hyperplasia, leading to mucus production and cough, and the obstructive disease, probably resulting from changes in the small airways, appear to be independent results of smoking.

In some patients, chronic bronchitis may be associated with such severe coughing as to produce hemoptysis. This must always be considered seriously, but if the sputum is merely blood streaked in association with exacerbation of cough and there are no associated lesions on the x-ray examination of the chest or careful physical examination of the lungs (Chapter 1), it is appropriate to ascribe the hemoptysis to bronchitis. The first episode of hemoptysis or expectoration of gross blood, particularly in the absence of heavy coughing, requires a complete evaluation, including bronchoscopy, in order to exclude a carcinoma of the lung. The smoker with bronchitis is also at high risk of developing lung cancer.

In most patients, the x-ray film of the chest will reveal thickening of the walls of the airways, pictorially termed tramlines by the British. These findings are not distinctive, since they are also present in asthma. In some patients, the bronchi are actually dilated, and the distinction between bronchial dilation associated with bronchitis and bronchiectasis is quantitative rather than qualitative. In addition, the enlarged openings to the mucus glands may be visible on bronchography as small pits or diverticula.

Bronchitis is characterized by periodic exacerbation of symptoms, sometimes associated with purulent sputum. These have been shown to be most commonly due to nonbacterial infections, though occasionally bacterial infections may be present and require treatment.

The differential diagnosis of chronic cough is not always straightforward. The new development of cough requires careful physical and x-ray examination to exclude parenchymal disease of the lung, especially tuberculosis. As discussed in Chapter 2, some patients with asthma may complain principally of cough, but they should also complain of chest tightness, and they should reveal airway obstruction relieved by bronchodilators or airway obstruction induced by exercise. On physical examination, patients with bronchitis frequently have rhonchi due to partial obstruction of airways, principally by mucus, but these rhonchi should change with cough and be present throughout the lungs. A localized audible or palpable rhonchus suggests an obstructing tumor, and an expiration film may reveal localized hyperinflation of the lungs.

Treatment

Obviously the treatment of chronic bronchitis is prevention by elimination of cigarette smoking. If this is impossible, an annual measurement of FEV_1 and demonstration of deterioration may aid the physician in convincing the patient that problems are in store and that smoking must be stopped. It has been shown that prophylactic administration of broad-spectrum antibiotics is associated with some decrease in the severity and duration of exacerbations of bronchitis, particularly in the winter, but it does not reduce the incidence of exacerbations. It is probably more practical to utilize antibiotics, such as 1 gm of tetracycline per day, when cough increases with increasing expectoration of purulent sputum. The Gram stain and cultures of the sputum are of little value in dictating the choice of therapy. Exacerbations of bronchitis, even if proven to be related to infection, are not generally associated with permanent worsening of ventilatory function, and antibiotic treatment is of no value in preventing the development of COPD.

In some patients, symptomatic treatment of cough is requested, but this may be difficult. It is probably unwise to suppress cough with codeine because it is important to maintain maximal patency of the tracheobronchial tree by expectoration of obstructing mucus. There is little evidence that the many expectorants available to the physician are of real value in either changing the viscosity of sputum or promoting expectoration. This is certainly true of popular agents such as potassium iodide and ammonium chloride, and there are conflicting reports about the value of glyceryl guaiacolate. Some have claimed that sputum volume is increased and viscosity decreased with large doses of this agent, but others have found no such effects. There are also reports that glyceryl guaiacolate increases mucociliary clearance so that, if an agent is to be selected, this is probably the most rational one to use.

In the absence of obstructive pulmonary disease, there is no compelling indication for the use of bronchodilating drugs, although it has also been shown that these agents, particularly the beta-adrenergic drugs, do increase mucociliary clearance. In patients in whom there is episodic wheeze or dyspnea, bronchodilators are certainly indicated and the most rational approach is to use a long-acting beta-adrenergic agent such as metaproterenol by aerosol inhalation every 4 to 6 hours. The treatment of obstructive pulmonary disease will be discussed in more detail below.

BRONCHIECTASIS

Pathogenesis

Bronchiectasis is defined as permanent dilatation of the airways. In many instances the difference between bronchitis and bronchiectasis is quantitative rather than qualitative, since airway enlargement is characteristic of bronchitis, and it is not particularly important whether the patient is labeled as having one condition or the other. The airway enlargement may take various forms, ranging from the generalized cylindrical dilation related to chronic bronchitis to saccular outpocketings characteristic of more localized disease. There is destruction of the dilated airway walls, and there are inflammatory changes within the airways associated with the production of copious secretions. One of the striking features of bronchiectasis is marked expansion of the systemic collateral circulation to that area of the lung. The bronchial arteries, which normally provide the blood supply to the major airways, proliferate extensively in bronchiectasis for reasons that are not completely understood. This increase in the systemic circulation is important because it can lead to severe hemoptysis when the vessels become eroded.

There are many known causes of bronchiectasis. Airway obstruction by a tumor or foreign body is generally associated with bronchiectasis distal to the occluding lesion, and even though this may be extensive, it is completely reversible if the obstructing lesion is removed at an early stage. Both viral and bacterial pneumonia are commonly associated with bronchiectasis, which disappears several weeks after the infection has healed. It is for this reason that bronchograms must be interpreted with caution after an acute pneumonia. Chronic inflammatory and fibrosing diseases of the lungs are frequently associated with bronchiectasis. Healed necrotizing gram-negative pneumonia and lung abscesses often leave a distorted and tortuous dilated bronchial tree, which may be a source of recurrent infection. Most tuber- culous lesions that heal with scaring are associated with bronchiectatic changes of the airways, and bronchiectasis is common in sarcoidosis as well as in diffuse interstitial fibrosis of other etiology. Finally, bronchiectasis appears to be very common after heroin pulmonary edema. This may be related to increased traction on the walls of the airway from the stiff lung.

Cystic Fibrosis

Cystic fibrosis is a specific cause of bronchiectasis that must be considered in young adults with chronic cough and sputum production. With improving care, many children with this disease now live to adult life. The pulmonary manifestations result from the production of abnormally sticky mucus by the bronchial glands, leading to airway obstruction and ultimately to bronchiectasis. This is the counterpart of the abnormal mucus in the intestine, which causes the usual presenting complaint of steatorrhea. The diagnosis of cystic fibrosis is made by the presence of increased concentra- tions of salt in the sweat, and a sweat test should be performed in young adults with generalized bronchiectasis.

Right Middle Lobe Syndrome

Bronchiectasis is also a feature of the right middle lobe syndrome. In this condition the right middle lobe becomes atelectatic with associated dilata- tion and destruction of the large airways. It probably results from obstruction to the right middle lobe, often by hilar adenopathy which subsequently disappears, leading to atelectasis and permanent changes in the airways and parenchyma. The susceptibility of the right middle lobe to collapse is due to the fact that the segments of the right middle lobe are unique in that they contain very little surface adjacent to other segments of the lung. As a result, when a segmental bronchus is occluded, there is less opportunity for collateral ventilation from adjacent segments to maintain expansion of the alveoli distal to the occlusion. The right middle lobe syndrome is generally detected, usually unexpectedly, when an x-ray film of the chest reveals opacification and contraction of this portion of the lung. It is often of little clinical significance. Recurrent infection or even bleeding is usually a minor problem, and the measures outlined below for the treatment of bronchiectasis, primarily postural drainage and antibiotics, are quite satisfactory. As with other forms of bronchiectasis, surgery is rarely necessary.

Bronchiectasis may also result from a genetic defect, and it is commonly found in congenital lesions such as sequestration of the lung, an abnormality related to the development of the lung in infancy. An unusual form of bronchiectasis is seen in asthmatics with mucoid impaction and aspergillosis. Only the central bronchi are dilated and the distal branches are normal, which is opposite to the findings in usual bronchiectasis.

Bronchiectasis may also occur without clear antecedent cause. It has been related to childhood infection of the lung, particularly with whooping cough or with some other form of bronchiolitis, and in all likelihood it represents the permanent sequela of acute inflammatory disease.

Clinical Features

Patients with bronchiectasis are frequently entirely asymptomatic, particularly if the disease is localized and the result of a previous infection. The most important symptom is chronic cough, generally associated with purulent sputum, which may be even foul-smelling in some cases. Inspiratory crackles are often present over the affected lung, as are rhonchi and, occasionally, wheezes. Clubbing of the fingers is a common finding in patients with diffuse bronchiectasis, and it is possible that the same factors that lead to expansion of the bronchial collateral circulation to the lung cause the increased circulation to the digits to produce clubbing. X-ray film of the chest may reveal the lesions causing the bronchiectasis or, in cases of diffuse disease, frequently shows increased bronchovascular markings.

It must be emphasized that precise diagnosis requires bronchography, and in some cases the plain x-ray may actually be normal despite bronchographic evidence of extensive disease (Fig. 3–1). However, bronchography is not indicated in the majority of patients. One can infer the presence of bronchiectasis in patients with evidence of a good deal of inflammatory disease and scarring on x-ray, and there is no need to delineate the extent of the lesion. In right middle lobe syndrome, the demonstration of bronchiectasis is of no particular consequence and even in diffuse bronchiectasis the distinction between bronchitis and bronchiectasis is unimportant. It is only when one contemplates surgery that bronchography becomes important, because it is essential to make sure that adjacent segments of the lung are free of disease if resection is to be carried out.

The clinical importance of bronchiectasis is largely dependent upon complications. The dilated airways with excessive production of mucus and loss of mucociliary transport are prone to recurrent infection, which must be identified and treated. Chronic obstructive pulmonary disease is frequently associated with diffuse bronchiectasis, as it is with bronchitis. Hemoptysis is a very important complication, which is generally more frightening than

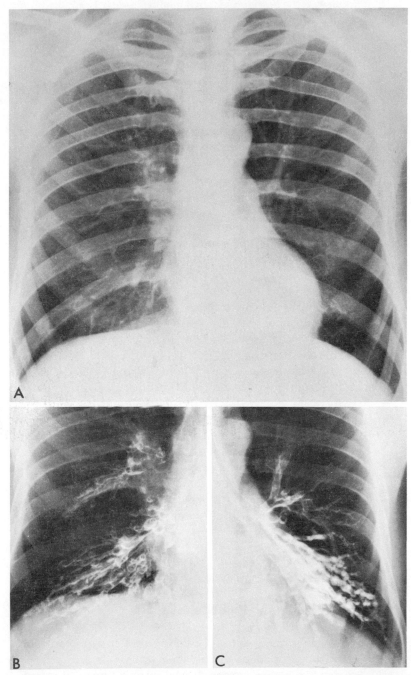

Figure 3-1   Bronchogram *(B* and *C)* reveals severe bilateral lower lobe bronchiectasis in a patient with little abnormality on the PA film of the chest *(A)*. (Reproduced with permission from Fraser, RG, and Paré, JAP: Diagnosis of Diseases of the Chest. 2nd edition. Philadelphia, W. B. Saunders Company, 1979, p. 1448.)

serious. Hemoptysis is particularly apt to occur during periods of active infection or in association with heavy coughing. As with bronchitis, blood streaking associated with heavy cough is of little consequence, and proper treatment with antibiotics and postural drainage generally serves to prevent or minimize this complication. Rarely, a large bronchiectatic air space richly endowed with collateral circulation may produce significant pulmonary hemorrhage; if this persists or occurs recurrently, it may require surgical treatment. A final, very rare complication of bronchiectasis is left ventricular failure due to the marked increase of collateral circulation, which represents a hemodynamic flow burden to the left ventricle. There are reports of individuals with left ventricular failure due to this cause which disappeared after surgical removal of the bronchiectasis.

Treatment

With improved medical therapy, bronchiectasis has largely been converted from a surgical to a medical disease. Indeed, the incidence of the condition has become markedly reduced in recent years as a result of the introduction of antibiotic therapy for pulmonary infections, and it is the rare patient whose symptoms are so severe that resection is required. The major principles of therapy are the use of postural drainage and antibiotics. Patients should be taught to adopt a position that will drain the bronchiectatic lobes at least twice a day in order to minimize stagnation of secretions and thereby prevent infection and progressive disease. A broad-spectrum antibiotic should be administered during periods of exa   at   n, which are reflected in increased cough productive of purulen   .um. If this is done, most patients will remain relatively well with   p gression of obstructive pulmonary disease or the development of severe hemoptysis. Repeated or continuing infections are one indication for surgery. If they occur despite good medical treatment in a patient with disease that has proven to be localized by bronchography, lobectomy may be indicated. Life-threatening hemoptysis that persists despite medical therapy may require emergency lung resection, and repeated bouts of hemorrhage despite intensive medical therapy with antibiotics and postural drainage are also an indication for resection.

EMPHYSEMA

Definition and Pathogenesis

Emphysema is defined as abnormal enlargement of the air spaces accompanied by destruction of alveolar walls. It is primarily a pathological lesion, but it may have important clinical implications. Like bronchiectasis, emphysema is associated with a wide variety of pulmonary lesions. These include inflammatory disease, such as tuberculosis; scarring in the lung, with retraction of adjacent air spaces, as in pulmonary fibrosis; and partial occlusion of a branch of a bronchus, with distal emphysema.

Extensive emphysema has two major variants. Centrilobular emphysema refers to the lesion that occurs in the center of the secondary lobule around a small airway and is most commonly associated with chronic bronchitis and bronchiolitis. It is probably related to the inflammatory changes in the airways that produce the obstructing pulmonary disease and also cause the alveolar destruction. It is more common in the upper than lower lobes of the lungs, and it is often found in patients with COPD but probably is of relatively little importance either as a cause of airway obstruction or in the management of the patient. Panacinar emphysema is extensive destruction of the entire lobule. It is most often found in the lower lobes of the lungs, and it is the type of emphysema associated with the most pronounced destruction and hyperinflation.

Emphysema may result from traction from adjacent lung, from the inflammatory destruction of lung tissue, or from the irritant action of air pollutants on small airways. There is little doubt that cigarette smoking is an extremely important cause of emphysema. The lesion has been produced by cigarette smoke in animals, and the vast majority of patients who have emphysema are or have been heavy cigarette smokers. There are many ways in which cigarette smoke might contribute to the development of emphysema. The irritant action on the airways, with production of excessive secretions, coupled with inhibition of mucociliary transport known to result from cigarette smoke may predispose to airway obstruction and inflammatory changes in the alveoli, particularly around the very small airways. In addition, it has been found that the alveolar macrophages from smokers produce excessive amounts of elastase in tissue culture and that cigarette smoke interferes with the inhibition of elastase. This enzyme may be active in smokers and cause dissolution of the elastic framework of the lung. In recent years, it has been recognized that individuals with deficiency of the serum globulin alpha$_1$ antitrypsin are particularly prone to development of emphysema. It is likely that this and other circulating proteins are necessary to protect the framework of the lung from proteolytic digestion resulting from activation of polymorphonuclear leukocytes and macrophages in any type of pulmonary inflammation or injury.

Clinical Features

Localized emphysema, often a single bulla visible on the x-ray film of the chest, is generally not associated with symptoms or with abnormal physical findings. Rupture of a bulla may lead to pneumothorax or pneumomediastinum. Progressive enlargement of a bulla may be associated with so much compression of normal lung as to produce symptoms, particularly in patients with diffuse obstructive airways disease, and an occasional patient may experience marked relief of dyspnea from surgical removal of the bulla.

Generalized emphysema is important in relationship to chronic obstructive pulmonary disease. There are two major ways in which emphysema can contribute to airway obstruction. Alveolar destruction may be associated with loss of the tethering action of lung parenchyma on the airways, which is important in maintaining patency of the airways. More important, loss of the lung elastic structure leads to loss of lung recoil so that the effective driving pressure for expiration, which stems from the increased alveolar pressure consequent to lung inflation, is markedly reduced. It is this loss of lung recoil pressure that contributes to airway closure, leaving unopposed the action of positive pleural pressure during forced expiration to compress the airways. It has been shown experimentally that emphysema is associated with some obstruction to expiratory flow rate, but generally this is relatively mild. In addition, there have been many patients with extensive emphysema and marked loss of lung recoil who have evidenced relatively little airway obstruction, so that emphysema is probably a minor rather than a major contributor to obstructive airways disease.

Generalized emphysema can be suspected from physical and radiographical examination but not with great precision. It is associated with an increase in total lung capacity, because of alveolar destruction, reflected in the hyperinflated lung evident on physical examination as a barrel chest and on the x-ray as hyperinflated lung fields. Similar findings, however, may be present in other types of obstructive lung disease, particularly in children with asthma who have marked degrees of hyperinflation without any alveolar destruction at all. Fairly accurate estimation of the severity of generalized emphysema can be obtained from pulmonary function studies. Alveolar destruction means that there has been loss of the alveolar capillary surface area available for the diffusion of gases, and this is reflected in a reduction of the diffusing capacity of the lung for carbon monoxide. In addition, the alveolar destruction is associated with loss of lung elastic recoil, and this is reflected in a pleural pressure that is less negative than normal. When the lung is inflated to a given lung volume, the intrapleural pressure, measured as eosphageal pressure in the pulmonary function laboratory, is less negative than normal. Radiographic examination may be of some additional value in outlining the extent of emphysema. Tomographic studies may better reveal decrease or absence of lung vessels, which generally signifies the presence of emphysema; angiographic study may be even more revealing in localizing the disease (Fig. 3–2). Thus, it is possible to obtain some evidence of the extent of emphysema, but this is of little consequence to the management of the patient and is of more academic than practical significance.

An interesting variant of this condition is *unilateral emphysema,* a condition associated with obstruction to the small airways in only one lung. It probably results from widespread broncheolitis in childhood. The lung becomes overexpanded and hyperlucent with a decrease or absence of the pulmonary circulation on angiography. Unless associated with contralateral disease, this condition is perfectly compatible with good health.

Treatment

There is no medical treatment for emphysema, though every effort should be made to prevent the condition by eliminating cigarette smoking. In some patients alveolar rupture from localized blebs or bullae may require pleural decortication to induce symphysis of the lung against the chest wall and prevent recurrent pneumothorax. As mentioned before, a small number of patients with increasing enlargement of localized emphysematous lung may benefit dramatically from surgical resection. The best candidates for such

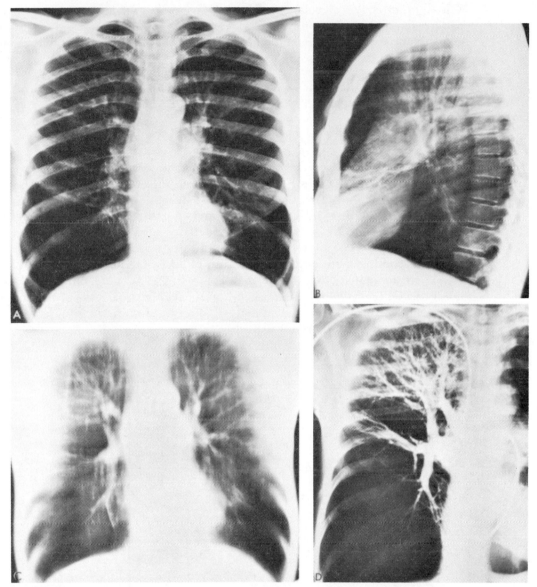

Figure 3–2 PA *(A)* and lateral *(B)* films of the chest reveal marked overinflation of the lungs with decreased vasculature suggestive of emphysema in the lower lobe. Tomogram *(C)* and angiogram *(D)* more clearly demonstrate the loss of vessels characteristic of emphysema. (Reproduced with permission from Fraser, RG, and Paré, JAP: Diagnosis of Diseases of the Chest. 2nd edition. W. B. Saunders Company, 1979, p. 1391.)

surgery are individuals with localized emphysema, and it is important to demonstrate that the lesion is compressing adjacent lung, with narrowing and crowding of airways and vessels best demonstrated on angiographic examination. Attempts have been made to treat generalized emphysema with surgical resection, based on the idea that if emphysematous lung is removed, the adjacent lung will be placed under increased stretch, thereby enhancing its elastic recoil pressure so as to improve expiratory flow rates. This follows from the argument that reduced expiratory flow rates are due to a loss of effective alveolar pressure as a result of loss of lung recoil. Experience with such treatment has been largely unsatisfactory, though an occasional patient with lower lobe emphysema has shown benefit following lobectomy.

CHRONIC OBSTRUCTIVE PULMONARY DISEASE (COPD)

Definition and Pathogenesis

COPD refers to that very large group of patients in whom chronic dyspnea is the result of generalized airway narrowing, often associated with emphysema. The mechanics responsible for the obstruction to expiratory flow are illustrated in Figure 3–3. COPD has become an extremely common cause of both disability and death, in direct proportion to the increasing consumption of cigarettes. Like lung cancer, it was once a disease of elderly males, but is now becoming increasingly common in older women.

There are many, often interrelated factors that contribute to the development of COPD. Probably the most important feature is disease of the small airways, the bronchioles. Inflammatory changes and narrowing of these airways are the most constant features, along with excessive secretions, in

NORMAL

COPD

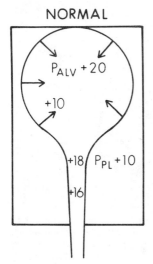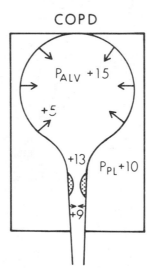

Figure 3–3 Mechanisms of expiratory obstruction in COPD. In the normal subject, the positive alveolar pressure (20) is the sum of the elastic recoil pressure of the distended lung and the positive pleural pressure generated by expiratory effort. The turbulent flow through the airways causes the pressure to drop from 20 to 16, but this is still higher than the pleural pressure, so that the airways remain patent.

In COPD, the lung recoil pressure is reduced because of emphysema, so that the effective pressure causing expiratory flow, the alveolar pressure, is only 15. In addition, there is a larger pressure drop down the narrowed airways, with the result that a point is reached at which the intraluminal pressure is less than the pleural pressure and flow stops. The loss of recoil pressure (emphysema) and the airway obstruction, singly or together, cause flow limitation such that, beyond a point, increasing pleural pressure by increasing expiratory effort no longer causes increase of expiratory flow rate.

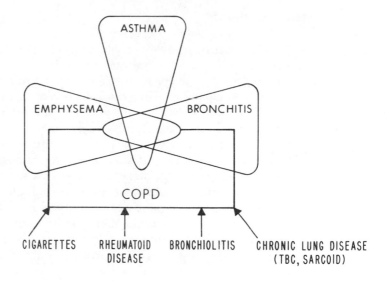

Figure 3–4 COPD may be associated with asthma, bronchitis, and emphysema singly or in any combination or, rarely, with none of them. Specific factors known to cause COPD include cigarette smoking, rheumatoid disease, acute or chronic bronchiolitis, and chronic lung diseases such as tuberculosis and sarcoidosis.

patients dying with COPD. It is now known that cigarette smoking causes narrowing of the small airways, reflected in sensitive tests of pulmonary function, and this may be reversible if cigarette smoking is discontinued at an early stage. This will be discussed below in relationship to the natural history and evolution of the condition. It has been reported that patients who have experienced an acute, extensive bronchiolitis, as from the inhalation of noxious chemicals such as ammonia, nitrogen dioxide, or chlorine, then develop chronic obstructive pulmonary disease. COPD is commonly associated with chronic bronchitis, though the majority of patients with bronchitis do not have it, and it is likely that the irritant pollutants that produce bronchitis also produce changes in the small airways, leading to the chronic obstruction. (See Figure 3–4.)

As noted, COPD is commonly associated with emphysema, again in all likelihood because of common etiological agents, but in some cases the emphysema may be the dominant cause of the airway obstruction. This is particularly true in patients with homozygous alpha$_1$ antitrypsin deficiency in whom severe emphysema may be the major cause of the obstructive pulmonary disease. In some patients with asthma the obstruction becomes relatively constant and irreversible. Thus, there are a great many factors that can produce the condition: chronic bronchoconstriction, excessive secretions in the airways related to both increased production and decreased clearance, narrowing and obliteration of the small airways, and emphysema.

Chronic obstructive pulmonary disease has also been associated with a number of other pulmonary diseases. Extensive tuberculosis is commonly associated with COPD, probably a reflection of the fact that tuberculosis frequently involves the airways, with consequent narrowing and obliteration. Likewise, it has been recently recognized that airway obstruction is a common feature of sarcoidosis, owing to the fact that sarcoid granulomas are often present in the airways, particularly late in the disease. An unusual form of rapidly progressive COPD, due primarily to bronchiolitis but without any emphysema, has recently been reported in patients with rheumatoid arthritis and other types of connective tissue disease. Finally, there have been case reports of COPD following an episode of acute diffuse lung disease.

Natural History

Aside from occasional reports relating COPD to a specific disease or event, there is little clear understanding of how it actually develops. It is known that the majority of smokers with bronchitis do not develop COPD, and serial studies of such patients have rarely revealed the development of serious airway obstruction. Individuals with a rapidly declining expiratory flow rate have generally been shown to have asthma.

Three possible pathways to COPD are suggested in Figure 3–5. It is possible that, in some patients, smoking is associated with a more pronounced decline of expiratory flow rates in the few patients who develop COPD than in the population at large (Line 2). On the other hand, it has been shown by retrospective study of patients who ultimately develop COPD that the course of the disease was not gradually progressive but, rather, characterized by a period of rapidly declining ventilatory function followed by relatively slow progressive impairment once the disease was established (Line 1). Supporting evidence for this theory is the fact that most patients with established COPD show very little progression from year to year. This is important because patients can be reassured that with continuing follow-up they will probably not get very much worse. Why the condition develops with such acceleration at the beginning and then tapers off is entirely unclear. Which of these two hypotheses represents the true pathway to COPD is not terribly important, but in either case it is important to follow smokers with serial measurements of expiratory flow rates so that any decline, be it slowly progressive or of sudden onset, can be detected and the patient warned that COPD is very likely to develop. A third possibility is represented by Line 3. There is evidence that patients with COPD very commonly had respiratory infection in childhood and that almost 50 per cent of smokers who have had a childhood respiratory illness are at risk of developing COPD. It is quite possible that acute childhood illness, probably a diffuse bronchiolitis, leads to widespread airway narrowing, which only

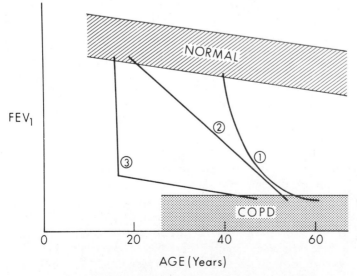

Figure 3–5 Potential pathways to COPD. (1) A smoker experiences rapid, then slower decline, of ventilatory function but then stabilizes with severe airway obstruction. Such a course has been described in a number of patients. (2) A smoker experiences a gradual decline of ventilatory function over 30 years until COPD is present. (3) Respiratory infection in a child (it could occur in an adult) produces marked but asymptomatic obstruction of airways followed by the decline in expiratory flow rates over several years expected in a smoker until COPD is present.

becomes symptomatic as obstructive pulmonary disease later in life. A similar event could occur in adult life with the abrupt development of airway obstruction.

As mentioned, it is now clear that cigarette smokers are very apt to have abnormalities of small airways detected on sensitive tests of pulmonary function, and these can become reversed if smoking is stopped. It is not clear that these abnormalities correlate with the subsequent development of COPD, but continuing studies of patients with these tests of pulmonary function may ultimately shed light on the evolution of this important condition.

Clinical Evaluation

A careful history can provide important clues regarding the cause, nature, and severity of COPD. Particular attention must be focused on the type and severity of dyspnea. Its onset, whether it is or is not associated with infection, either sudden or gradual, and any related complaints are particularly important. It must be remembered that dyspnea is a subjective complaint, and there have been many documented instances of patients with severe airway obstruction who were free of symptoms and who only complained of dyspnea after some acute illness or pneumonia. Respiratory infection may focus the patient's awareness on symptoms previously disregarded, and although pneumonia has often been cited as the cause of ensuing COPD, there are very clear data indicating that in patients with bronchitis and with COPD neither intercurrent infections nor episodes of ventilatory failure are associated with permanent worsening of ventilatory function. Episodic dyspnea, particularly associated with wheeze, may suggest a diagnosis of asthma, and chronic cough is strong evidence of associated bronchitis. Smoking history and other evidences of air pollution, in the home or in industry, are important clues to etiology. A history of childhood respiratory illness suggests that a patient is particularly at risk of developing COPD, and a patient with rheumatoid or other connective tissue disease may have the particularly virulent form of bronchiolitis, which is known to be rapidly progressive and usually fatal.

In patients with established disease, ankle swelling may be an indication that cor pulmonale has developed and careful inquiry must be made regarding signs of ischemic heart disease, such as angina pectoris or a previous myocardial infarction, in order to evaluate the possibility of left ventricular failure as an independent complication. As described in Chapter 1, critical inquiry must be made in order to separate paroxysmal dyspnea originating with left ventricular failure from the worsening dyspnea that occurs sometime after lying down in patients with chronic obstructive pulmonary disease.

Physical examination can often suggest the presence of COPD. Pursed-lip breathing, hyperinflation of the chest, use of the accessory muscles of respiration, impaired diaphragmatic function, and rhonchi have been described in Chapter 1. The roentgenogram is essential to exclude other diseases of the lung parenchyma and may provide suggestive leads to diagnosis, such as hyperinflation, areas of hyperlucency, suggesting emphysema, or increased bronchovascular markings, which are characteristic of bronchitis but also occur in chronic asthma.

Evaluation is dependent upon pulmonary function studies, and the presence and severity of COPD are best reflected in measurements of forced expiratory flow rates. These tests do not provide definitive information about the type of obstructive disease that is present, though impairment of expiratory flow rates (FEV_1) and FEF25-75% in the presence of a normal or even increased vital capacity strongly suggests that emphysema is a major component. Asthma is suggested by a marked response to bronchodilators, but the variability of that test has been emphasized in Chapter 2. Changes in FEF25-75% may be misleading if there is significant change of vital capacity. In most patients, vital capacity is terminated by the need to take another breath. If the forced expiration is prolonged, the calculated FEF25-75% will fall because more of the tracing contains the very slow, terminal expiration than is the case when expiration is interrupted early. For this reason, FEV_1 is a more satisfactory index of changes in airway obstruction. It is independent of the depth of the expiration. In addition, patients often find it difficult to make a prolonged, full expiration.

Other tests of lung function may be obtained for the evaluation of patients with COPD, but they are of more academic than practical value. An increased total lung capacity is strongly suggestive of emphysema, as is reduction of diffusing capacity and of lung recoil force. Patients may have normal spirometric findings and still have small airways disease only detectable by specialized tests such as measurement of closing volume, flow volume curves, frequency dependence of lung compliance, or a comparison of the flow volume curve during air breathing to that obtained with helium breathing. These tests are of interest in population studies and shed more light on the evolution of COPD, but they are of little practical value, since the significance of small airways disease is not firmly established as a prelude to COPD, although it probably is. Patients symptomatically short of breath from obstructive pulmonary disease will certainly reveal reduced expiratory flow rates, and severe disease is associated with an FEV_1 of 1 liter or less.

Patients with advanced COPD develop hypercapnia and hypoxemia, both of which require arterial blood gas analysis for assessment. Hypercapnia is due to inadequate ventilation in relationship to metabolic rate and largely reflects the increased work of breathing through obstructed airways. There is variability in this relationship, and some patients with hypercapnia have decreased activity of the respiratory centers, hypoventilating at a level of obstruction that is associated with an adequate ventilation in others. This becomes a very important factor in the management of patients hospitalized with COPD but is of relatively less importance in outpatients. Hypoxemia is primarily the result of differing ventilation/perfusion ratios in the lung, since some units receive much more blood flow than ventilation and contribute hypoxemic blood to the arterial circulation. This too is of major consequence to hospitalized patients, and provides the basis for and guide to oxygen therapy, but is not necessarily a required measurement in the ambulatory patient. The management of ventilatory failure is discussed in Chapter 9.

Treatment

Unfortunately, the treatment for COPD is largely supportive, and although a great many drugs and techniques have been utilized, they are of very limited value.

Table 3-1 Treatment of COPD

Bronchodilators — beta-adrenergic aerosol and theophylline by mouth
Promote cough — position, clapping; guaiacolate
Antibiotics — for infection
Breathing exercises — rapid inspiration, passive expiration
Condition — by progressive exercise
Oxygen — during sleep
Corticosteroids — if documented increase of FEV_1
Psychological support — antidepressants
Surgery — resection of compressing bullae
Diuretics — for congestive heart failure

Bronchodilators

Bronchodilators are certainly useful in patients with a reversible component demonstrated on spirometric study. Since both beta-adrenergic agents and, probably, theophylline enhance mucociliary clearance, these drugs are often given to patients with COPD on a regular basis. One can give theophylline and an adrenergic agent such as metaproterenol every 6 to 8 hours, as for asthma, or utilize the adrenergic agent as an aerosol, which is probably more effective and without side-effects. If this is done, one should employ metaproterenol at intervals of 4 to 6 hours in order to maintain a continuing effect. The effects of isoproterenol are so short lived as to be of little value unless given frequently.

Secretion Reduction

Chronic cough is often a major problem in patients with COPD, and secretions, which constitute an important component of airway obstruction, should be dealt with as effectively as possible. Some patients respond to postural drainage with effective expectoration, and it is worthwhile having the patient assume the various positions that will enable drainage from the different segments of the lung in order to learn whether or not one or more positions are associated with increased expectoration. If so, postural drainage should be carried out in this fashion two or three times a day. As discussed in connection with bronchitis, there is no firm evidence that available drugs are effective in facilitating expectoration, but if an expectorant is to be used, the most rational agent is glycerol guaiacolate. Some physicians have patients inhale mists and vapors in an effort to liquify the sputum, but there is no evidence that this type of treatment is actually effective. Hydration is often used to promote expectoration, but there is also no evidence that it is effective. Cough suppression is probably not wise, except in patients with a totally dry cough in whom the irritation of cough may produce bronchoconstriction and worsening obstruction, as in asthma. If this is the case, small doses of codeine may be useful. It is worthwhile for the physician to listen to the patient cough. Audible sounds of secretions in the large airways suggest that vigorous measures should be pursued to improve tracheobronchial clearance. Of course, the most effective way to decrease cough is to stop smoking.

Antibiotics

It has been shown clearly that antibiotics are of little value either in improving pulmonary function or in affecting the natural history of COPD. Nonetheless, recurrent bacterial infections are not uncommon, and most physicians prescribe a broad-spectrum antibiotic, without sputum examination, for episodic worsening of cough and expectoration of purulent sputum.

Breathing Exercises

Many types of breathing exercises have been developed and used in patients with COPD, but there are really no data indicating that such exercises actually improve pulmonary function. Attempts have been made to restore diaphragmatic excursion by encouraging the patient to protrude the abdomen during inspiration, and this is a rational approach to the dyspnea associated with overinflated lungs. The most sensible type of breathing exercise is based upon the nature of the airway obstruction. In patients with COPD, maximal expiratory flow rate is achieved with very little expiratory effort, and forced expiration is associated with, if anything, decreasing flow and a notable increase in the work of breathing, which may be interpreted as dyspnea. It is for this reason that many patients adopt pursed-lip breathing. It prevents the airway compression which limits flow, so that when they do perform a maximum expiratory effort they at least maintain flow rate. It is more rational to teach the patient not to make a forced expiratory effort but to breathe in as rapidly and actively as possible and, then, to allow the lungs to empty passively in order to minimize expiratory effort and airway closure. Active inspiration increases the time available for expiration, thus promoting lung emptying and improving ventilation. This type of exercise, plus abdominal breathing and postural drainage, can be taught easily by the physician or, if available, a respiratory therapist.

Progressive Exercise

Some centers have advocated progressive exercise as a means of improving the physical working capacity of patients with COPD. Although the patient can increase tolerance to exercise, both in intensity and in duration by progressive exercise, as on a treadmill, the evidence shows that this is not associated with measurable improvement of lung function. Nonetheless, such an approach does increase activity and may improve the quality of life, so that a program of graded exercise, easily accomplished by encouraging the patient simply to walk increasing distances twice a day, may be useful. In some patients, exercise tolerance can be improved by oxygen breathing, and portable oxygen may be used as an adjunct to this treatment.

Intermittent Positive Pressure Breathing

For many years intermittent positive pressure breathing (IPPB) was used in the treatment of patients with obstructive pulmonary disease. There is a good deal of evidence now that such treatment has no effect on lung function, that it does not enhance the effectiveness of aerosol bronchodilators delivered by freon nebulizer, and that it is of no long-term benefit with respect to morbidity or mortality. There are occasional patients with severe dyspnea who claim to experience marked relief from IPPB and it may be useful in such instances, but it is probably of more psychological than physiological value. Some patients have difficulty using cartridge nebulizers and may benefit from bronchodilators delivered by IPPB or other mist generators.

Chronic Oxygen Therapy

The recent availability of portable liquid oxygen cylinders has made it more practical to use chronic oxygen therapy in patients with COPD. There is evidence that such treatment, in hypoxic patients, reduces pulmonary artery pressure and prevents polycythemia and attendant congestive heart failure. There is recent evidence that this treatment actually prolongs life.

Attention has also been directed to the possibility that oxygen may be given only during the night with considerable benefit. Recent studies have shown that most patients with COPD experience episodes of profound hypoxemia during sleep. The mechanism of this is not entirely clear, but it is prevented by inspiration of low concentrations of oxygen. It is possible that maintenance of normal arterial oxygen tension during sleep may have a favorable influence both on psychological function and on prevention of the complications of congestive heart failure. Before embarking on chronic oxygen therapy, the physician must demonstrate the presence of hypoxemia, and it is best to institute the therapy in the hospital to be sure that there is no severe suppression of ventilation by the treatment. It can then be carried out at home, utilizing nasal prongs and the administration of oxygen from either a conventional tank or a portable oxygen cylinder. Chronic oxygen therapy may also increase mobility of patients who become hypoxic during exercise, and if this is the case, portable oxygen from a liquid oxygen cylinder may be useful.

Corticosteroids

Corticosteroids have been utilized in a great many patients with COPD, and in most reports it is the occasional patient who responds with improved expiratory flow and symptoms. One clue to such a beneficial response is the presence of eosinophils in the sputum; patients with physiological evidence of advanced emphysema are much less likely to respond. Nevertheless, there have been occasional patients who seemed to have severe emphysema who responded to corticosteroid therapy; and it is probably worthwhile to embark upon a therapeutic trial in patients with severe symptoms, particularly in the presence of sputum eosinophilia. Such a trial should be done very carefully and should include measurements of expiratory flow rate before and after steroid therapy. If there is no improvement of expiratory flow rate, the treatment should be stopped; even if the patient experiences symptomatic relief, the hazards of steroid therapy are only outweighed by the demonstration of physiological improvement. To date, the steroid aerosols have not proven to be of benefit in patients with COPD, but only a limited number of patients have been treated. Aerosols require more careful evaluation and can be given to individual patients as a therapeutic trial in conjunction with appropriate spirometric testing.

Psychological Support

The psychological support of the concerned physician is of great importance in the management of the patient with COPD. These individuals are, for good reason, frequently depressed, but it is possible to reassure the patient that with appropriate management the disease need not progress and that symptoms will not necessarily worsen. It has been shown that, in some instances, the intensity of dyspnea is correlated with psychological depression, and there may even be a role for antidepressive medication in addition to an attitude of cheerful optimism in the treatment of these patients.

Surgical Treatment

A variety of surgical approaches have been used for the treatment of COPD. There is a small number of patients with localized emphysema in whom resection of a bulla that is compressing adjacent normal lung can lead to dramatic improvement. Beyond this, attempts at treatment of diffuse lung disease by lobectomy or other surgical measures have not proven very satisfactory.

Tracheostomy

Chronic tracheostomy has been performed on patients with advanced COPD but is probably indicated only very rarely. It has been suggested that reduction of the dead space by tracheostomy might reduce ventilatory requirements and, hence, the severe dyspnea. This is not the case, since the marked increase of physiological dead space because of $\dot{V}/\dot{Q}$ abnormalities is little affected by the small decrease of anatomic dead space achieved by tracheostomy. Patients who have required prolonged intubation for artificial ventilation may need a tracheostomy until they can be weaned from the respirator, but it is now known that one to two weeks or even longer of endotracheal intubation can be tolerated, and conversion to tracheostomy may be delayed until it is evident that a prolonged period of artificial ventilation will be required before the patient can resume spontaneous ventilation.

Tracheostomy has also been advocated as a means of aspirating secretions from the tracheobronchial tree, but it should be emphasized that cough is the most effective means of promoting airway clearance. Mechanical suction is of principal value in patients who are unable to cough by themselves. In patients with upper airway obstruction, and this may be a complicating problem in obese patients with COPD, tracheostomy may be a very important means for providing unimpeded breathing during sleep. Finally, performance of a chronic tracheostomy may be useful in that it generally discourages cigarette smoking. In general, however, tracheostomy is now used for continuing ventilator management, and chronic tracheostomy is only indicated in patients with upper airway obstruction or in patients with such recurrently frequent ventilatory failure as to require almost constant treatment with a respirator.

COMPLICATIONS

Congestive Heart Failure

Congestive heart failure has been shown to be primarily a consequence of hypercapnia and hypoxemia. Correction of the latter by chronic oxygen therapy and improvement of obstructive disease with improvement of ventilation and lowering of Pco_2 are the major measures used to prevent the development of pulmonary hypertension and right-heart failure. In patients with edema, a low-salt diet and diuretics are extremely useful. The weight of evidence suggests that digitalis is not of value in this condition, that right ventricular function is not improved in these patients, and that unless coexistent left ventricular disease is present digitalis probably should not be used. This is particularly the case in patients hospitalized with ventilatory failure in whom the dangers of arrhythmia are already present and apt to be accentuated by digitalis.

The physician must follow patients with COPD with great care, searching for signs of congestive failure so as to intensify treatment and utilize diuretics; identifying worsening cough, which may respond to antibiotics or postural drainage along with chest percussion; and treating other reversible components, such as bronchoconstriction, as thoroughly as possible. In addition, attention should be paid to the environment and air pollution reduced to a minimum. Not only the patient but all those who enter the home should be forbidden to smoke, and patients working in a dusty occupation may even have to change their job. With due care, most patients with COPD can be treated at home most of the time; in fact, there is little done in the hospital that is not available to the patient in the home.

Surgery

Like everyone else, patients with COPD may develop illness requiring surgery, and the physician is often called on to evaluate such a situation. It is known that patients with COPD are at much greater risk of complications from any type of surgery than patients who are free of cough and dyspnea. But it has also been shown that if such patients stop smoking prior to therapy and embark on a regular regimen of bronchodilator therapy associated with breathing exercises and prophylactic antibiotics, the risk of complication becomes very much less. In fact, serious complications are not common, and the patient with severe COPD who requires surgery can certainly have it. If an elective procedure is contemplated, more post-operative difficulty is anticipated in these patients, but the risks do not prohibit the surgery. It should be borne in mind that, during surgery, patients are managed with artificial ventilation, just as they would be treated for ventilatory failure, so that there is little risk during the procedure itself. It is the postoperative atelectasis, pneumonia, ventilatory failure, and related complications that must concern the physician. These can be minimized by appropriate measures designed to encourage cough and deep breathing and to prevent infection.

General surgery is not associated with worsening of obstructive pulmonary disease. In contrast, thoracic surgery requires much more careful study and although the guidelines are not entirely clear, one useful principle is to consider that surgery can only be performed if the resultant FEV_1 will be 600 cc or better. One can estimate this by measuring ventilatory function, assessing the contribution of the diseased lung to be resected by ventilation-perfusion scans of the lung and, then, estimating what the post-resection pulmonary function will be. Patients with severe airway obstruction associated with hypercapnia at rest are probably not candidates for resectional surgery, but other patients can be evaluated in this way.

CASE REPORT

The following case report, reprinted with permission from the *New York State Journal of Medicine,* illustrates many of the features of COPD.

This is the description of a patient who endured a severe form of COPD (chronic obstructive pulmonary disease) for several years. He demonstrated remarkable improvement after tracheostomy, only to die shortly thereafter of a pulmonary embolus. He illustrates many common features of the pathogenesis, pathophysiology, and natural history of COPD and some features that are less common. The response to tracheostomy demonstrates the important role of upper-airway obstruction in some patients and, in addition, promotes speculation about the role of the respiratory center in this condition.

Pathogenesis and Natural History

During childhood, the patient experienced two types of illness which may have contributed to the COPD which developed in his forties. He had mild asthma, never requiring hospitalization and disappearing in his teens. It is known that most patients with asthma do not develop emphysema, but many adults with asthma do have relatively chronic airway obstruction, and an asthmatic component is often present in patients with COPD. It is also known that most patients with asthma do not smoke cigarettes, but the patient began smoking very heavily in his youth, two to three packs a day right up to near the end of his life. It is possible that his self-indulgence, in contrast to the meticulous avoidance of all pollution characteristic of most patients with asthma, represents the rather unusual complication of constant irritation from cigarette smoke to abnormally reactive airways and, hence, the eventual COPD. In addition, he had pneumonia three times as a child, and there is evidence that in many patients, COPD is the result of bronchiolitis, perhaps occurring as one or more discrete events, and that the injury is present long before the symptoms become evident or disabling. It appears that the combination of widespread small airways injury from acute infection, the abnormally reactive airways of asthma, and the constant irritation from cigarette smoke set the stage for what was to come.

When he was 42 years old, the patient began developing shortness of breath and wheeze which soon became so severe that he gave up his job as a construction worker and went to work as a chauffeur. The symptoms worsened, and six years later, when he was 48, he had to give up this job and spend his days at home. This was very difficult because he was an active man, proud of his strength and ability to support his family. His main joy was derived from his work and from sociability. He enjoyed parties and all that was left now was the continuing cigarette habit. During the next two years he was admitted three times to a veterans' hospital for severe CO_2 (carbon dioxide) retention and, on each occasion, he required endotracheal intubation, an event that was to occur repeatedly thereafter in our own hospital.

In 1973, when he was 50 years old, he was first brought to the emergency room of the Bronx Municipal Hospital Center unresponsive and cyanotic, with signs of congestive heart failure. His arterial Pco_2 (carbon dioxide pressure) was 90 mm Hg, his Po_2 (oxygen pressure) was 36 mm Hg, and his oxygen saturation was 67 per cent. He quickly became comatose and was intubated, placed on a ventilator and, after a few days, the endotracheal tube was removed and he was sufficiently improved so as to be able to go home. This was the first of 29 admissions to the Bronx Municipal Hospital Center, monotonously similar in nature, with initial presentations of varying degrees of somnolence and asterixis responding to therapy with or without intubation.

Pulmonary function studies were first performed in 1973 and revealed severe airway obstruction with fairly substantial response to bronchodilators, confirming the historical data suggesting an asthmatic component to the condition (Table 3–2). Total lung capacity was normal; the reduced diffusing capacity and Pmax (pleural pressure) both suggested the presence of emphysema. Subsequent measurements of vital capacity and FEV_1 (forced expiratory volume) obtained during hospitalizations all revealed values less than those obtained as an outpatient in the pulmonary function laboratory, and, at least on one occasion, December, 1973, there was substantial improvement of the obstruction during hospital treatment. It is noteworthy that exacerba-

Table 3–2 Pulmonary Function Studies

Tests	VC* (liters)	FEV_1† (liters)	TLC‡ (liters)	Dco§ (ml per min, mm. Hg)	Pmax‖ (cm H_2O)
Normal	4.3	3.3	6.4	31	21
September, 1973	1.7/2.6	0.4/0.7	6.6	16	16
December, 1973	0.9–1.5	0.4–0.6	—	—	—
January, 1974	0.7	0.3	—	—	—
September, 1974	0.6	0.3	—	—	—
October, 1974	0.8	0.3	—	—	—
March, 1975	1.5/1.8	0.4/0.4	6.6	6	11
December, 1975	0.5	0.3	—	—	—
April, 1976	0.9	0.4	—	—	—
November, 1976	1.3	0.3	—	—	—

*Vital capacity before/after bronchodilation.
†First forced expiratory volume in one second.
‡Total lung capacity.
§Diffusing capacity for carbon monoxide.
‖Negative intrapleural pressure at total lung capacity.
Other measurements of VC and FEV_1 were obtained on the ward during hospitalization, and the values noted on December, 1973, represent the range from admission to discharge.

tions and worsening of ventilatory failure were not associated with marked reduction of FEV_1, a common finding in patients with COPD in whom worsening is not readily explained by increased airway obstruction, but rather is the culmination of a series of vicious cycles involving airway obstruction, hypercapnia and hypoxemia, polycythemia, pulmonary vasoconstriction, salt and water retention, and pulmonary congestion. In March, 1975, the airway obstruction was a little worse, but noteworthy is the fairly marked drop of diffusing capacity and Pmax. This suggests progression of pulmonary emphysema, subsequently confirmed to be extensive at postmortem examination. It is interesting that the worsening emphysema was not associated with much decrease of expiratory flow rate, emphasizing the relative unimportance of emphysema as a cause of airway obstruction. It is now known that extensive emphysema can be present with only trivial airway obstruction, and the obstruction in COPD is much more the result of changes in the airways: inflammation, scarring, and particularly, secretions. It is also interesting that, in this patient, the emphysema worsened over a 2-year period, whereas many of the patients we have followed showed no such change over up to 10 years of followup. Progression is more the exception than the rule. Patients and their physicians should understand quite clearly that COPD and emphysema are not necessarily inexorably progressive.

Ventilatory Failure and Response to Tracheostomy

The patient's 29 admissions to the Bronx Municipal Hospital Center are sketched in Figure 3–6, which is a plot of the highest arterial P_{CO_2} and the P_{CO_2} at the time of discharge on each occasion. These represent a fraction of the blood gas measurements obtained during this time, and the arterial P_{CO_2} was usually well over 50 mm Hg. Noteworthy is the fact that a great many episodes of ventilatory failure were successfully managed without intubation, and on many occasions medical therapy was effective when the arterial P_{CO_2} was over 100 mm Hg. Therapy over these years consisted of oral bronchodilators, theophylline (Elixophyllin), inhalation of isoproterenol, and intensive efforts to help the patient raise the copious, thick secretions which were present most of the time. Needless to say he was constantly urged to stop smoking. Because some patients with COPD respond to corticosteroids, particularly if they have sputum eosinophilia, the patient received prednisone for several months, but there was no definite evidence of improvement. Likewise, some patients with alveolar hypoventilation, particularly if they are obese, may experience increase of alveolar ventilation when treated with progesterone. A trial of this drug was also ineffective. In 1974, we talked to the patient about performing a tracheostomy. We felt that this was indicated to obviate the need for recurrent intubation, that it might make it possible for him to aspirate secretions more effectively, and that it might also make him stop smoking. This was suggested at each admission; each time he gave it thought, but always decided that he would go home to try once more. The usual pattern was that he would return home with a P_{CO_2} in the 50s, remain well for a few days to a few weeks, and then start smoking heavily out of aggravation, boredom, and despair. Eventually, however, the patient did stop smoking in March, 1975, and he stopped for good. Noteworthy is the fact that for several months he no longer had to come into the hospital and managed to fend for himself at home. This is a dramatic illustration of the role cigarettes played even at this late stage of the disease. Nonetheless, the effect was short lived, and he finally returned again in the usual fashion.

These admissions illustrated another dramatic but common adaptation. Frequently the arterial Po_2 was 20 mm Hg and this, in the face of a concentration of carboxyhemoglobin of from 10 to 20 per cent from the heavy smoking, represents a lethal degree of hypoxia when experienced acutely. In patients with COPD, chronic hypoxia is associated with polycythemia, increase of cardiac output, possibly rightward shift of the oxyhemoglobin dissociation curve to promote oxygen release to the tissues and, most importantly, increased tissue capillarity so that oxygen can reach the cells even when present at a very low partial pressure in the blood. The patient was well acclimatized to chronic hypoxia.

During these admissions another component of his illness became evident. Asterixis and somnolence were a prominent feature of his course, but the somnolence did not always correlate with the degree of CO_2 retention. During the past few years it has been noted that, in obese patients, somnolence and hypercapnia do not correlate, and that upper airway obstruction is a major problem. Upper airway obstruction develops during sleep, leading to prompt and frequent arousal. Sleep deprivation is the major cause of the somnolence. Upper airway obstruction has also been noted in nonobese patients and is not an uncommon complication of intubation-induced damage to the large airways. It was noted that the patient developed stridorous respiration during sleep, that respiration became very shallow or even ceased, and that sleep was punctuated by periods of arousal with restoration of normal breathing. We considered the possibility that abnormality of the respiratory center was playing a role in the hypoventilation, and for three nights he slept in a Drinker respirator. This resulted in sleep at night and, the next morning, an arterial Pco_2 far below that which it had been in the past (Fig. 3–6), but the respirator was so uncomfortable that he soon gave it up.

The dominant features of somnolence and asterixis coupled with the evidence of upper airway obstruction during sleep added new impetus to the consideration for tracheostomy. Thus, in addition to treating secretions, we might remove a major contributor to the hypercapnia by establishing a patent upper airway. Finally, in September, 1976, the patient consented. Tracheostomy was performed and after a few days the respirator was removed and, for the first time in over three years, the arterial Pco_2 became normal and remained so. Figure 3–6 illustrates this correction of hypercapnia but underestimates the phenomenon. Actually, multiple blood gas determinations were in the normal range with a Pco_2 usually 36 to 42 mm Hg. Coincident with this, there was a dramatic change. The patient became bright, alert, and enthusiastic. He was ambulatory, and his newly found enjoyment in life was evident to all. For two weeks he still demonstrated irregular respiration during sleep, but a month after the tracheostomy his respiration was normal and regular at all times. This leads to the speculation that the chronic hypercapnia had some effect on the respiratory center so as

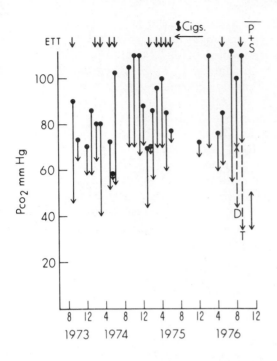

Figure 3-6 Highest and final arterial Pco_2 recorded during admissions; small arrows signify endotracheal intubation performed. P + S signifies recurrent pneumothorax leading to thoracic surgery; D represents arterial Pco_2 following use of Drinker respirator, and T indicates tracheostomy.

to produce diminished and irregular respiration, particularly during sleep, which only disappeared after several days to weeks of eucapnia. This might be similar to the reversible loss of chemoreceptor response in patients with chronic hypoxia who regain their hypoxic stimulus to breathing after correction of hypoxemia. Noteworthy is the fact that CO_2 breathing two weeks after the tracheostomy did not produce any increase of ventilation, indicative of an abnormal respiratory center. We believe that tracheostomy produced an immediate improvement by by-passing upper airway obstruction, but that continuing improvement of respiration was related to a gradual return of respiratory center function to normal after the hypercapnia was corrected.

The Final Irony

With his return to health, the patient was ready to go home and he was discharged only to face a new series of problems. His returning strength and activity led to new expectations from both himself and his wife, and this apparently resulted in such anxiety that he returned to the hospital once again with shortness of breath. But this time his blood gases were normal and, with reassurance, his symptoms disappeared. We decided that we would help him gradually return to a normal life by discharging him for short periods and enable him to make the transition back to health gradually. This was not to be. In November, 1976, he suffered the first of three spontaneous pneumothoraces. Is it possible that the increased expansion of the emphysematous lung during normal respiration, made possible by the tracheostomy, resulted in increased stress and strain so as to cause alveolar rupture? Noteworthy is the fact that, despite almost total collapse of the right lung, he remained free of hypercapnia and on no occasion did the Pco_2 rise over 45 mm Hg. The pneumothoraces were treated by chest tube, and, finally, when collapse persisted and it became evident that the lung would not expand, he had a thoracotomy with successful resection of an emphysematous bulla, insertion of chest tube, and expansion of the right lung. Once again he improved, remained eucapnic off the respirator, but suddenly on the seventh postoperative day he was found dead in bed. In addition to severe emphysema, autopsy revealed a massive pulmonary embolism.

During the final hospitalization, there was a sense of inevitability and irony in that this patient, who was disabled at a relatively young age with severe respiratory insufficiency, was on the road to restoration of health, only to experience new disability from pneumothorax and, when that was successfully treated, a fatal embolus It is as if the outcome were written in advance and resolution of one problem was inevitably followed by another, perhaps in some way a result of the previous success.

Additional Reading

Brashear RE, Rhodes WL: Chronic obstructive lung disease. St. Louis, C. B. Mosby, 1978.
Cherniack RM, Lertzman MM: Management of patients with chronic airflow obstruction. Med Clin North Am 61:1219–1228, 1977.
Fletcher C, Peto R, Tinker C, Speiger FE: The Natural History of Chronic Bronchitis and Emphysema. New York, Oxford University Press, 1976.
Thurlbeck WM: Chronic airflow obstruction in lung disease. Philadelphia, W. B. Saunders, 1976.

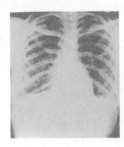

CHAPTER FOUR

PULMONARY INFECTIONS

Pulmonary infections represent a large component of the practice of the primary physician. There is a broad spectrum of disease, extending from mild upper respiratory infection to acute, fulminant bacterial pneumonia and the chronic indolent disease associated with tuberculosis. A proper diagnosis is extremely important so that appropriate therapy can be applied as early as possible and, almost equally important, so that unneeded antibiotics will not be given. The physician must rely heavily upon the bacteriology laboratory, especially for the final, accurate diagnosis, but in many instances prompt therapy is so important that it should be based upon the physician's own examination of the sputum smear.

TUBERCULOSIS

Once the province of the phthisiologist, then the chest physician, tuberculosis is now the concern of the general internist and primary care physician. This is the result of the fact that successful chemotherapy has made it possible to treat many patients at home, at least during most of their illness, so that there is no longer a need for specialized facilities. In addition to treating the illness, which occurs in a great many forms, physicians must be familiar with the pathogenetic features of tuberculosis, so they can carry out their responsibility for detecting and preventing the disease in the community.

Pathogenesis

Tuberculosis results from the inhalation of a droplet nucleus containing a viable *Mycobacterium tuberculosis*. Such droplet nuclei are generated as an aerosol by patients with active disease, particularly when they cough. It is now known that the order of contagion is very low. So few droplet nuclei are dispersed into a ventilated room that inhalation of contaminated air for many months is required before infection will result.

If a viable tubercle bacillus reaches the lung, it produces a mild inflammatory reaction in the periphery, usually in the basilar segments, which receive relatively more ventilation than the upper portions. The organism multiplies slowly but is disseminated through the lymphatics and the blood stream to many different areas of the body. There is, initially, very little inflammatory response, but when the T-lymphocytes become activated they produce an inflammatory response that serves to localize the tubercle bacilli at the various sites they have reached. At this time the tuberculin test becomes positive. In individuals with heavy bacteremia, disseminated miliary tuberculosis may develop as a relatively acute, virulent illness. This may either result from the initial bacillemia, with widespread dissemination of small lesions throughout the lungs and other organs, or develop later when a caseous focus ruptures into a blood vessel from trauma or for some other reason. Miliary tuberculosis is a particularly dreaded form of disease in infancy.

In over 90 per cent of individuals the infection is completely controlled, and disease never results. In a small percentage of individuals, particularly very young children or patients with an impaired immune response, active primary tuberculosis may develop. This is generally manifest as an inflammatory lesion in the lung, which may be as large as a lobar pneumonia, with a characteristic enlargement of the draining hilar lymph nodes. In another, probably equally large group of patients, reactivation tuberculosis may develop at a later time after the initial infection. This is most apt to occur during the first two to three years, about half the cases appearing at this time. It is for this reason that conversion of the tuberculin reaction is a major indication for chemoprophylaxis. Reactivation, or reinfection, tuberculosis most commonly develops in the upper portion of the lungs. This is because the apices receive relatively more ventilation than perfusion than other portions of the lung so that the oxygen tension within the alveoli is high. This produces a very favorable condition for the growth of the aerobic tubercle bacillus.

Adult infection is characterized by progressive inflammatory reaction with caseous necrosis and, ultimately, breakdown, with the formation of cavities. At this stage of the disease dissemination occurs by continuing aspiration of infected sputum to different parts of the lung. This bronchogenic spread leads to inflammation, caseation, and even further cavitation in other parts of the lung. Reactivation tuberculosis may also occur in any of the other organs that have been seeded by the initial bacillemia. Tuberculous meningitis, the result of a cortical tuberculous lesion rupturing into this meninges, is the most serious of these infections. Other common sites for infection include the kidney, bones, joints, lymphatic system, and serous membranes.

The reasons for the development of adult reactivation tuberculosis are not entirely clear, but there are a number of risk factors that are felt to be important. Any suppression of immune response, as with chemotherapeutic agents or corticosteroids, may be associated with the development of the disease. It is particularly common in the first few years after the initial infection; it is apparently more likely to occur in patients with poorly controlled diabetes than in others; it is unusually common, for reasons unknown, after gastrectomy; it is common in silicosis; and it is more likely to occur in individuals with visible lesions from the primary infection than in

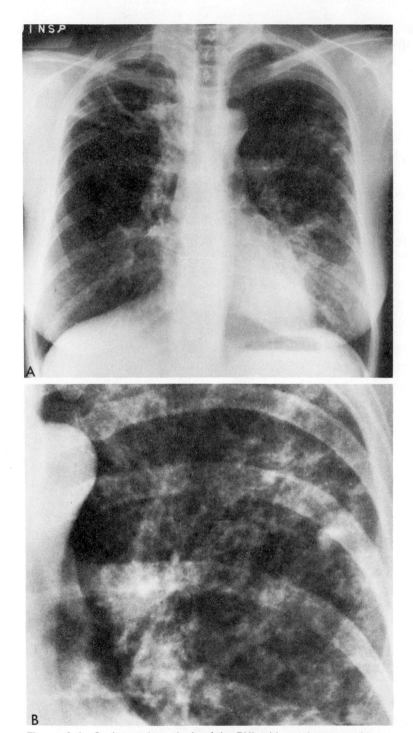

Figure 4-1   Cavitary tuberculosis of the RUL with patchy areas of bronchogenic spread to the left lung. (Reproduced with permission from
Fraser, RG, and Paré, JAP: Diagnosis of Diseases of the Chest. 2nd
edition. W. B. Saunders Company, 1979, p. 750).

those in whom the x-ray film of the chest is normal. All of these risk factors are important indications for isoniazid prophylaxis. In addition, there is a good deal of evidence that emotional factors are very important in the development of reactivation tuberculosis. It has been related to loneliness and grief, and it is particularly common among alcoholics. The development of tuberculosis after loss of a loved one has been repeatedly documented in art and literature and in clinical studies. In addition, prior to chemotherapy there were many instances of successful treatment of tuberculosis following improvement of the emotional state.

Clinical Features

Tuberculosis is a disease with such protean manifestations that it is impossible to do more than summarize some of the important clinical findings. It should be emphasized that tuberculosis remains very much a problem in the United States, particularly in urban areas, and it must always be considered in patients with chronic febrile illness. It is still one of the leading causes of fever of unknown origin.

Most patients are ill because of pulmonary infection. Primary tuberculosis is often associated with cough, fever, and mild constitutional symptoms. The roentgenogram usually reveals unilateral hilar adenopathy with a variable degree of pneumonic reaction at the primary site of infection in the lung. More commonly, the disease presents because of reactivation of the infection of the upper portions of the lung. Characteristically, symptoms are present for many weeks or longer, and they include malaise, fever, and cough. Some degree of hemoptysis is very common, particularly in patients who develop cavitation. The roentgenogram generally reveals many areas of infiltration in the lungs with one or more cavities. Usually one large cavity can be identified as the source of the initial caseous necrosis and breakdown that led to bronchogenic dissemination to other parts of the lung. Over 90 per cent of the patients have a positive tuberculin test, and the sputum contains *Mycobacterium tuberculosis*. Diagnosis requires identification of these organisms on acid-fast stain and, ultimately, culture, which is also necessary in order to determine the susceptibility of the organisms to antimicrobial agents so that appropriate therapy can be prescribed.

Miliary tuberculosis is a much more rapidly developing, usually more serious acute illness manifest by fever and evident infection in various organs. Choroidal tubercles are an important physical finding. Meningitis is a common complication and must be evaluated by lumbar puncture, with measurement of spinal fluid protein and glucose as well as acid-fast stain and culture. Tuberculous pleurisy will be discussed in Chapter 7. Less frequently the disease may present as peritonitis with ascites or as pericarditis. Tuberculous arthritis is a not uncommon form of monarticular arthritis; tuberculous osteomyelitis, most frequently involving the spine, can lead to severe thoracic deformity. The kidneys are often affected by the tubercle bacillus, often asymptomatically in patients with disease evident in the lungs. In some individuals the disease is confined to lymph nodes. Cervical adenitis is a common form of tuberculosis in children, and there is often no evidence of disease in the lungs. Tuberculosis may be associated with a variety of hematological reactions, including various types of myeloid metaplasia as well as severe anemia. In all cases the diagnosis must be established by identification of tubercle bacilli in the infected organs.

Pulmonary lesions exhibit great variability on radiologic examination. They include pneumonic consolidation or even a diffuse interstitial lesion resulting from hematogenous dissemination. Miliary tuberculosis usually is characterization by uniform small nodules, but a similar appearance can be produced by many other diseases. Tuberculosis must be considered in any patient with radiographic abnormalities of the lung, and diagnostic efforts must be pursued until the organism can be recovered or another diagnosis established. Reinfection disease is not always confined to the upper lobes, and diabetics are particularly prone to develop the disease in the lower lobes. If the patient does not have cough productive of sputum, it is wise to obtain three morning gastric aspirates for culture for tubercle bacilli. The gastric contents may contain other acid-fast organisms and the tubercle bacillus frequently is not evident on smear, so that this technique is only useful as a source of positive cultures that take from six to eight weeks. In addition, sputum can be induced by the inhalation of hypertonic saline by aerosol for smear and culture. In difficult cases, fiberoptic bronchoscopy with bronchial and transbronchial biopsy may be needed to establish the diagnosis. It must be emphasized that although 90 per cent of patients with active tuberculosis have a positive tuberculin test, some do not, and a negative tuberculin test does not absolutely exclude the diagnosis.

Treatment

The essential feature of the treatment of tuberculosis is effective chemotherapy. The most effective drugs are isoniazid, ethambutol, rifampin, and streptomycin. All of these agents have profound antimicrobial effects, but since any population of tubercle bacilli is apt to contain mutants that are resistant to at least one of these drugs, treatment with any one of them may be followed by improvement, with subsequent, progressive disease due to resistant organisms. For this reason, at least two effective drugs must always be used for the treatment of tuberculosis; patients with severe disease such as miliary tuberculosis are given three drugs.

Isoniazid (INH) is always used in the initial treatment of tuberculosis, and in most instances the companion drug is ethambutol because of its efficacy and very low toxicity. If more drugs are needed, rifampin should be included, and if there is any doubt that the patient will continue to take therapy for several months, rifampin should be the companion drug to INH. Chemotherapeutic agents should be administered daily at least for several months and until the x-ray film has stabilized and sputum cultures and smears are negative for tubercle bacilli. It is then wise to continue therapy for an additional twelve months for maximal eradication of the disease and prevention of subsequent relapse. A variety of alternative regimens have been advocated in order to shorten the period of treatment, but it is not entirely clear that these regimens are satisfactory; it is safer to continue with regimens that have been proven to be effective. There is evidence that isoniazid and ethambutol can be administered in larger doses twice a week instead of every day, but there is no great advantage to this therapy in most patients. It should be remembered that if the patient on less than a daily regimen forgets to take a dose of the drug, the effects will be more serious than if a daily dose is omitted.

Treatment should be started when the diagnosis is first established by positive smear, and if the subsequent cultures reveal that the organism is resistant to one or more of the agents initially selected, two drugs to which the organism is sensitive must then be added. Even if the organism appears to be resistant to isoniazid, it is wise to continue to administer this drug because there is some evidence that the INH-resistant organisms, which are usually catalase-negative, are relatively inactive and much less likely to produce disease than the INH-sensitive catalase-positive organisms. However, the catalase-negative organisms may multiply, with development of mutants that are pathogenic, and may cause spread of disease unless isoniazid is given. There is evidence that patients with chronically active disease and positive sputum reveal little or no progression as long as isoniazid is given, even though the organisms in the sputum are resistant to isoniazid.

With therapy, one can expect disappearance of constitutional signs and symptoms within a short period of time, generally within a month and, then, slow but progressive improvement of the roentgenogram. In some patients the improvement is slower. On occasion progression of the disease or even the development of new diseases, such as a pleural effusion, may appear during the first six weeks of treatment. This does not require a change of the drug regimen. Pulmonary infiltrates should diminish or disappear; cavities should become smaller; and after several months the x-ray, although often abnormal, will become stable, indicating that the inflammatory disease has been controlled, with only residual fibrosis remaining. In patients with extensive disease, fibrosis may be considerable and is almost always associated with bronchiectasis, which may be a source of superimposed bacterial infection or of hemoptysis in the future. The development of fever and pulmonary infiltrates at the site of an old tuberculosis lesion is more likely a result of superimposed infection than reactivation of the disease. Tuberculosis may heal with persistence of cavities, which is designated the open-negative syndrome. Cystic airspaces may remain for years without causing difficulty. They may become infected with bacteria or with aspergillus in the form of a fungus ball, and these infections may be complicated by hemoptysis, but the cavities are not likely to be a source of reactivation of tuberculosis. They should be treated as any cystic airspace on the basis of the complications that arise.

The chemotherapeutic agents all have the potential for toxicity. Isoniazid may be associated with peripheral neuritis, particularly among alcoholics, and such individuals should probably receive pyridoxine to prevent the vitamin B_6 deficiency induced by INH. A substantial number of patients receiving isoniazid develop an increase of serum transaminase levels during therapy, but in most individuals the abnormalities revert to normal despite continuing treatment. A small percentage of patients do develop hepatitis, and when this occurs, the drug should be stopped. Hepatitis is much more common in older people, increasing at age 35 and over. It is very rare in people younger than 35.

Ethambutol is probably the least toxic of the therapeutic agents. Although it can cause optic neuritis in high doses, in the recommended dosage this complication is virtually nonexistent. Rifampin is the newest drug and is one of the most effective of the new drugs available for the treatment of tuberculosis. It is much more costly and slightly more toxic than isoniazid. It is associated primarily with liver toxicity and a variety of hypersensitivity reactions, including fever, rash, and purpura. Rifampin and methadone induce the metabolism of each other in the liver, so that addicts maintained on methadone may experience withdrawal symptoms when treatment with rifampin is started, requiring an increase in dose. Streptomycin is the oldest of the effective agents developed for treatment of tuberculosis. It is useful in patients with organisms resistant to the three major drugs or in patients with drug reactions to these agents, but the disadvantages are that it must be given intramuscularly and is associated with eighth nerve and renal toxicity.

A great many other drugs are available for the treatment of tuberculosis (Table 4–1). None of them is as effective as the first line drugs, but they are of great value in patients with organisms resistant to the primary agents.

The major problem associated with effective chemotherapy for tuberculosis is the continuing administration of effective drugs for as long as they are necessary. For a great many reasons patients often do not take the medicine prescribed, and continuing surveillance by the physician is absolutely essential. If therapy is interrupted, as often occurs among alcoholics or individuals with severe emotional problems, one can expect an exacerbation of tuberculosis, and in this case it may be due to organisms that are resistant to the primary therapeutic agents. One must then select two agents to which the organism is sensitive and reinstitute therapy with these drugs. One of the most important principles of retreatment is never to add a single drug at a time. At the very least, two effective new agents must always be given in order to prevent emergence of resistant organisms.

Table 4–1 Chemotherapy for Tuberculosis

Drug	Daily Dosage	Side Effects
PRIMARY DRUGS		
Isoniazid	300 mg PO	Peripheral neuritis, hepatitis, hypersensitivity
Ethambutol	25 mg/kg PO for 60 days, then 15 mg/kg	Optic neuritis
Rifampin	600 mg PO	Hepatitis, hypersensitivity reactions
Streptomycin	1 g IM	8th nerve damage
SECONDARY DRUGS		
Viomycin	15–30 mg/kg up to 1 g IM	8th nerve damage, nephrotoxicity
Capreomycin	15–30 mg/kg up to 1 g IM	8th nerve damage, nephrotoxicity
Kanamycin	15–30 mg/kg up to 1 g IM	8th nerve damage, nephrotoxicity
Ethionamide	15–30 mg/kg up to 1 g PO	Gastrointestinal, hepatotoxicity hypersensitivity
Pyrazinamide	15–30 mg/kg up to 2 g PO	Hyperuricemia, hepatotoxicity
Para-amino-salicylic acid	150 mg/kg up to 12 g PO	Gastrointestinal, hypersensitivity, hepatotoxicity, sodium load
Cycloserine	10–20 mg/kg up to 1 g PO	Psychosis, personality changes, convulsions, rash

Poor complicance with therapy is closely associated with major psychological and social problems, such as alcoholism and drug addiction, which must be treated as effectively as possible. The availability of methadone treatment programs has greatly improved the outlook for addicts with tuberculosis, and these patients can receive their antituberculosis chemotherapy under supervision at the same time as they receive methadone.

Primary resistance to effective agents is extremely unusual but must be evaluated by determining the sensitivities of cultured organisms. In addition, there are a growing number of individuals who are infected with atypical mycobacteria. These organisms are extremely resistant to the therapeutic agents and generally require treatment with three or more drugs from the very beginning. Atypical infection does not respond to therapy as well as typical tuberculosis and is one of the few indications for primary surgical therapy.

Aside from treatment of associated medical problems such as malnutrition and anemia, the general measures that were once the mainstay of tuberculosis therapy are no longer felt to be important. It has been shown that bed rest offers no additional advantage over effective chemotherapy, and patients who are not acutely ill can be fully ambulatory. Corticosteroids have been shown to have a beneficial effect on tuberculosis, so long as they are administered in conjunction with chemotherapy, by rapidly reducing the inflammatory reactions to the disease. Steroids are associated with prompt decrease of temperature, more rapid improvement of x-ray lesions, and general return of well-being and increased appetite. However, it has been shown that this improvement is not associated with long-term benefit. After six months of therapy the results in patients treated with steroids are not different from the results in patients without steroids.

Steroids have been advocated under special circumstances, but the evidence for their value is inconclusive. Patients desperately ill with extensive tuberculosis are frequently given corticosteroids just to promote improvement as rapidly as possible, but there is evidence that this treatment does not have an effect on mortality. Steroids are generally given to patients with tuberculous meningitis in order to prevent the complicating meningeal scarring that may result from this disease. It has been shown that corticosteroids hasten the resolution of pleural effusion and the same may be true of tuberculous pericarditis, but there is no good evidence that the ultimate serosal scarring is prevented. In the absence of chemotherapy, corticosteroids prevent the inflammatory response to tuberculosis, which results in the localization of the disease. Thus, steroid therapy has been associated with the rapid development of disseminated tuberculosis, the symptoms often being masked by the steroids, and chronic steroid therapy is one indication for isoniazid prophylaxis. Certainly a trial of steroids in an ill patient should never be given without chemotherapy unless tuberculosis has been absolutely excluded as a diagnostic possibility.

Some patients are hospitalized during the initial period of diagnosis and treatment, but many others with milder disease are now treated at home from the beginning. It is clear that the institution of chemotherapy is rapidly followed by reduction and elimination of infectious organisms in the sputum, in part because isoniazid is excreted in the sputum to act on expectorated bacilli. It should be recalled that patients are only contagious to the extent that they aerosolize tubercle bacilli into the air. If they can be taught to cough into disposable tissues, they are at little risk to their contacts. A number of studies have shown that patients treated with chemotherapy are not apt to cause infection among their contacts. If the sputum does not contain acid-fast bacilli on smear, the patient is not likely to be a risk to others. It is now felt that the patient with active tuberculosis can be discharged to the home within two to three weeks of institution of therapy, even if the sputum continues to be positive, and that patients without a positive smear can be treated at home from the beginning.

Tuberculosis laryngitis is the one indication for strict isolation. It has been shown that this complication, which can result from prolonged exposure of the larynx to heavily positive sputum, is, in contrast to all other forms of tuberculosis, a highly communicable disease. Patients with tuberculosis who are hoarse must have a laryngeal examination, and if tuberculous laryngitis is present, they must be kept isolated until treatment has been effective. These patients should be kept in a room with adequate circulation and ultraviolet lights, which have been shown to keep the air relatively free of infectious particles, and attendants should wear masks for their own protection.

Prevention

In addition to treatment of the patient with tuberculosis, physicians have a major responsibility in their own practice and community to prevent the development of disease in others. The contagious patient must be placed on continuing therapy, with precautions about coughing as noted previously. In addition, individuals seriously at risk for developing tuberculosis, particularly of a virulent sort, must be identified and placed on isoniazid prophylaxis. One year of therapy has been shown to decrease substantially the number of cases of active tuberculosis among people at risk. This requires a careful search for contacts, primarily in the household. Infants and young children associated with a patient with active disease should all be placed on isoniazid immediately, and if the tuberculin test is negative in three months, the drug can be stopped. Other household contacts with a positive tuberculin test should also be treated after radiographic examination to exclude active disease, which would require therapy with two rather than one drug.

Other people particularly at risk of developing tuberculosis should also be given isoniazid prophylaxis. Since isoniazid is virtually nontoxic in individuals less than 35 years of age, all such people with a positive tuberculin test are advised to take a year of treatment. Older patients with any of the risk factors noted previously — recent conversion, silicosis, steroid or immunotherapy, gastrectomy, and particularly evidence of old disease on x-ray — should also receive isoniazid prophylaxis. Surveillance for INH toxicity is maintained by monthly contact with the patient for symptomatic evidence of hepatitis, such as anorexia, nausea, vomiting, or dark urine.

Tuberculin Test

Since the tuberculin test is pivotal in the evaluation and control of tuberculosis, it is important to describe the proper way to perform this test. The proper
reagent is the intermediate dilution of PPD (5TU) This must be injected
intracutaneously, not utilizing the multiple puncture technique, and the
reaction should be measured as millimeters of induration at 48 hours.
Although one cannot induce sensitivity by repeat testing, it is known that
individuals with a minimal reaction will have a booster effect from the test,
which is evident within one week and lasts for over a year. Thus, a weakly
reactive patient at initial testing might have a positive reaction several
months later, because of the booster effect of the first test, which would be
falsely interpreted as a tuberculin conversion. To avoid this problem, and to
confirm the tuberculin status of the patient, a second tuberculin test is given
one to two weeks after the first. If positive, there is no point in further
testing, and a judgment as to the need for isoniazid would be based on age
and the presence of other risk factors. If the second tuberculin test is
negative, the test can be repeated annually as a screening measure in children or among individuals in a community where the disease is prevalent.

PNEUMONIA

Pneumonia continues to be a major health problem in the United States and,
despite the use of antibiotics, an important cause of death. It ranges from a
mild illness associated with a small infiltrate on the x-ray film of the chest to
progesssive, extensive involvement of the lung leading to death. The most
critical diagnostic step is isolation of the infecting organism from sputum,
from blood, or even from the lung in order to provide specific, effective
antimicrobial therapy.

Certain aspects of the history are extremely important in making the
initial decisions about management. In an otherwise healthy patient with
fever and cough, a pulmonary infiltrate is much more likely to be pneumococcal pneumonia than any other type of infection. In contrast, patients who
have recently been in the hospital or who have been in nursing homes where
other patients have received antibiotics are likely to be infected with some
other organism, and they may even require treatment with broad-spectrum
antibiotics in the absence of definitive bacteriological diagnosis. Patients
on corticosteroids, immunosuppressed patients, or patients with underlying disease are very much at risk of infection with unusual organisms and
probably should be hospitalized for proper treatment. If pneumonia develops
in a setting of epidemic respiratory infection the likelihood of a mycoplasma
or viral illness is high.

Patients acutely ill with high fever, with extensive involvement of the
lung on x-ray, or patients with severe associated disease or those on drugs
that predispose to serious infection must be hospitalized. Other patients
can be treated as outpatients, and although every effort should be made to
examine the Gram stain of the sputum, in many instances this does not
reveal a definitive organism. In such circumstances, the most appropriate
therapy is erythromycin, on the assumption that the pneumonia is of bac-

terial origin, such as a pneumococcus, which would be sensitive to the drug, or that there is a mycoplasma infection, which is also treated by this agent.

Patients hospitalized with pneumonia must be investigated with great care. In examining the sputum, one must make certain that the specimen is not from or heavily contaminated by oral secretions and one should only pay attention to a sputum smear that contains polys and macrophages and is free of buccal epithelial cells. If a sputum specimen cannot be obtained, it may be induced by inhalation of hypertonic aerosol, or it may be necessary to perform transtracheal aspiration. In seriously ill patients, it is also possible to perform percutaneous needle aspiration of the infected lung to be certain that the organisms revealed on Gram stain are those responsible for the pulmonary infection.

Pneumococcal Pneumonia

The pneumococcus is still the most common cause of pneumonia. It is most common in winter and spring. It starts by aspiration of organisms into the alveolar units of the lung and is often preceded by an upper respiratory tract infection or some other event, such as ingestion of alcohol, which impairs mucociliary clearance and favors deposition and retention of pathogens in the alveoli. The organisms multiply and rapidly provoke an inflammatory response, leading to exudation of edematous fluid, which then migrates through the pores of Kohn in the alveolar walls and through the air spaces into adjacent units of the lung, rapidly causing progressive inflammation. This proceeds through the stages of red and gray hepatization, and in treated or spontaneously resolving cases heals completely without residual damage. The infection is often adjacent to pleural surfaces, accounting for the high frequency of coincident pleural effusion and occasional empyema. The disease usually begins suddenly with fever and chills, cough productive of rusty or green sputum, and pleuritic pain. Inspiratory crackles are present in the affected areas, and there may be signs of consolidation. X-ray examination reveals an alveolar filling infiltrate, which may or may not have a lobar distribution. Incomplete consolidation of the pneumonic lesion is particularly apt to occur in patients with chronic pulmonary disease, such as emphysema, in whom the large air spaces fail to fill with the infected exudate. In some cases, the inflammation may spread from infected airways, producing a patchy appearance on the roentgenogram (bronchopneumonia).

Pneumococcal pneumonia, particularly of the lower lobes, may present many confusing features. It is not uncommonly associated with jaundice, apparently the result of hemolysis; and upper abdominal pain, often accompanied by paralytic ileus, may be so severe as to raise the question of acute cholecystitis or even peritonitis.

In hospitalized patients it is essential to obtain cultures as well as smears from the sputum, as outlined previously, and blood cultures. Sputum cultures are, disappointingly, frequently negative in patients in whom the Gram stain reveals gram-positive diplococci, and blood cultures may be the only source for precise identification of the organism. Sputum culture is much more likely to be positive if the specimen is promptly inoculated into the agar medium.

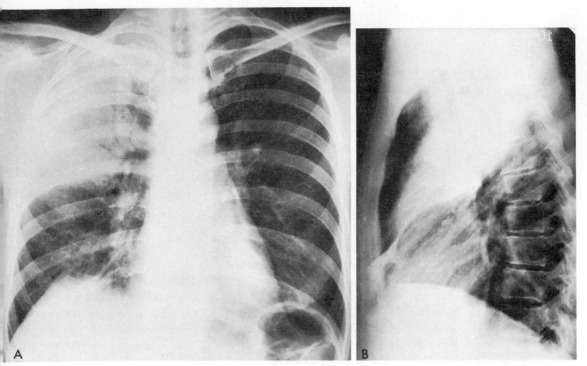

Figure 4–2 PA *(A)* and lateral *(B)* x-ray films of the chest in pneumococcal lobar pneumonia of the right upper lobe. Note the air bronchogram on the PA film signifying filling of alveolar spaces adjacent to unobstructed airways. (Reproduced with permission from Fraser, RG, and Paré, JAP: Diagnosis of Diseases of the Chest. 2nd edition. W. B. Saunders Company, 1979, p. 350).

There is an important subset of patients with pneumococcal pneumonia who are at extremely high risk, and the mortality is as high as 25 per cent. These are patients with significant underlying disease, leukopenia, extensive involvement by roentgenogram (more than one lobe of the lung), or a positive blood culture, alcoholics, and patients with diminished consciousness and inability to cough and expectorate infected secretions. Such patients should be carefully followed in an intensive care unit with monitoring of vital signs, careful replacement of fluids, and encouragement of coughing or, if necessary, frequent nasotracheal suctioning. Arterial blood gas tension should be measured. Although hypercapnia is rarely a problem, hypoxemia is common because of the abnormal ventilation/perfusion ratios in affected segments of lung. Nasal oxygen or oxygen through a venturi mask should be administered in sufficient concentration to maintain the arterial oxygen saturation at or above 90 per cent.

Penicillin is the treatment of choice and 600,000 units twice daily is sufficient. Larger doses should be avoided because of the possibility of the emergence of superinfection with penicillin-resistant organisms. Patients sensitive to penicillin may be treated effectively with erythromycin.

Treatment is usually followed by prompt decrease of fever and improvement of well-being. Failure to respond to treatment or the development of new symptoms requires careful search for superinfection. Pleural effusion commonly accompanies pneumonia; although it probably should be tapped initially to exclude empyema, it otherwise requires no specific therapy. Appropriate antibiotic therapy should prevent the development of such serious complications as brain abscess and meningitis. In healthy patients, the roentgenogram should clear within six weeks; in older patients or individuals with underlying lung disease there may be residual abnormalities that disappear very slowly. In such patients there is no need for x-ray examination more frequently than every six weeks, and one need not be concerned about residual lesions for up to four months.

The recent development of pneumococcal vaccines provides important prophylaxis for patients with chronic lung disease or for others who are at risk of developing pneumococcal infection.

Other Gram-Positive Pneumonias

Much less commonly, pneumonia is caused by staphylococcus and, rarely, streptococcus. Unlike pneumococcal pneumonia, these infections often lead to necrosis and destruction of lung tissue, with cavity formation and residual impairment of pulmonary function. Staphylococcal pneumonia is particularly common in association with epidemics of viral infection, especially influenza. It is usually associated with severe illness manifest as toxicity, chills, and high fever. The roentgenogram will reveal progressive infiltration, with abscess formation and, frequently, pleural effusion. Patients with this illness must be treated in a hospital with a penicillinase-resistant penicillin such as methicillin or oxacillin, preferably 2 grams intravenously every 4 hours. The effective therapy should be continued for at least 2 weeks. Streptococcal pneumonia is mainly confined to military populations in which streptococcal infection is common. It is usually associated with meningitis and is effectively treated with penicillin.

Gram-Negative Pneumonias

Infections with gram-negative organisms are particularly common in hospitalized patients or in patients from nursing homes that employ antibiotics widely in their patients.

Hemophilus influenzae

Hemophilus influenzae appears to be a particularly common cause of pneumonia among patients with chronic obstructive pulmonary disease or immune defects. It usually presents as multiple areas of bronchopneumonia on the x-ray, commonly associated with pleural effusion, but as in all other cases diagnosis depends upon isolation of the organism from uncontaminated sputum or pleural fluid. Since *H. influenzae* is present in the sputum of patients with COPD, its isolation is clinically significant only when it is the sole organism isolated from the sputum, preferably obtained through transtracheal aspiration. Like the pneumococcus, *H. influenzae* often fails to grow from the sputum culture. Ampicillin, 1 to 2 grams intravenously every 6 hours, is the treatment of choice, though sensitivity studies should be performed.

Klebsiella pneumoniae

Klebsiella pneumonia is a particularly serious gram-negative infection, often occurring in alcoholics, with a marked tendency to necrosis and abscess formation. The diagnosis may be suggested by the presence of bulging fissures on the x-ray film of the chest, and the organism should be identifiable in the sputum as a plump gram-negative encapsulated bacterium. Treatment with cephalothin or an aminoglycoside such as gentamicin is best dictated by the sensitivities prevalent in a given community.

Other Gram-Negative Organisms

Other gram-negative organisms such as *Pseudomonas* or *Proteus* may occur in the compromised host or hospitalized patient. Treatment depends upon identification of the organism and its sensitivity to antibiotics.

A major cause of gram-negative pneumonias has been the use of contaminated aerosols for the treatment of obstructive pulmonary disease. It is extremely important that if such equipment is used, it be frequently sterilized and monitored very carefully for bacterial contamination.

Legionnaire's Disease

In recent years an increasing number of patients with extremely virulent progressive pneumonia, first appearing in Philadelphia at an American Legion convention and therefore named Legionnaire's disease, have been identified. This illness is due to a gram-negative bacterium that is very difficult to grow in the laboratory but for which specific serologic and staining tests are now available. There is evidence that this organism is aerosolized from contaminated refrigerant units in large air-conditioning systems and that this was the source of the airborne infection in Philadelphia as well as in many other outbreaks, including epidemics in the New York City garment district and several hospitals. The disease is characterized by weakness, malaise, cough, and increasing fever, with relative bradycardia that is often of sudden onset. Hemoptysis is common and leukocytosis is the rule. Patchy infiltrates are evident on the roentgenogram, and they tend to progress rapidly. Other organ involvement with nausea, vomiting, gastrointestinal bleeding, and renal failure are common, and the mortality seems to be quite high. Erythromycin appears to be the treatment of choice and may cause dramatic improvement. Treatment should be continued for at least three weeks. Patients ill with progressive pneumonia, with unexpectedly severe hemoptysis and evidence of abnormal liver function, who come from an endemic area should be suspected of having this disease and should be treated with erythromycin. Serial serological studies should be performed to make a definite diagnosis.

Nonbacterial Pneumonia

Mycoplasma pneumoniae

Mycoplasma pneumonia accounts for most of the nonbacterial infections. The organism is transferred by droplet nucleus, and is often spread within families or associated with epidemics. It is usually associated with upper respiratory infection, with a variety of systemic symptoms and involvement of other organs. It may present as an interstitial pneumonia, characteristically less extensive than would be expected from the severity of constitutional symptoms, but the radiographic findings are not distinctive and may appear as lobular or lobar infiltrates. Mycoplasma pneumonia has been associated with severe respiratory insufficiency but is usually self-limited and mild. The roentgenogram should clear within two weeks if involvement is confined to a single lobe and within one month if more than one lobe is involved. Constitutional symptoms and chronic cough usually persist, even for several weeks after the acute infection, leading to the appropriate designation "walking pneumonia." The diagnosis is suggested by the absence of leukocytosis and the relative prominence of upper respiratory and constitutional symptoms without extensive involvement on x-ray. Cold agglutinins may be positive early in the course, and the physician can test for this by placing a specimen of citric-acid–anticoagulated blood in ice and noting the appearance, within a few minutes, of clumps of red cells as the tube is slowly tilted to allow the blood to flow down the side. Specific serological testing provides definitive diagnosis. Erythromycin or tetracycline is the agent of choice for treatment.

Viral Infections

Viral infections are very common among adults, but most cases of pneumonia are the result of infection with influenza and adenovirus. Influenza is most important as a prelude to the development of bacterial pneumonia, but primary influenza pneumonia can present as a very serious interstitial pneumonia and lead to adult respiratory distress syndrome and ventilatory failure. This usually develops rapidly with high fever, chills, and systemic symptoms, with progressive infiltrates on x-ray film of the chest. When influenza is complicated by bacterial pneumonia, the latter should be treated. Influenza vaccination is indicated for those at high risk of developing respiratory disease, such as patients with chronic obstructive pulmonary disease or chronic heart failure.

Unresolved and Recurrent Pneumonia

Failure of pneumonia to resolve, and this may take several months, requires a careful search for a predisposing factor such as carcinoma of the lung. Likewise, patients in whom pneumonia occurs more than once in the same location must be suspected of having serious underlying disease. This is usually bronchiectasis, but careful radiographic examination and, probably, bronchoscopy should be performed in these patients in order to exclude a tumor. Persistent pneumonia, particularly in the lower lobes, may be the result of chronic aspiration, as in patients with diaphragmatic hernia or in patients who ingest mineral oil. Lipid pneumonia may be confirmed by the presence of macrophages filled with vacuoles, from the sputum or bronchial aspirate, that stain positively with Sudan IV. Rarely bacterial pneumonia heals with extensive fibrosis and cholesterol deposition in the affected area, leading to the appearance of a mass lesion on x-ray. It is very difficult to exclude carcinoma in such cases, and on occasion the diagnosis can only be made by resection of the lesion.

It is not uncommon, particularly among patients with chronic lung disease, for cough and expectoration to persist some time after institution of appropriate antibiotic therapy. Sputum culture may soon reveal a new set of organisms, now resistant to the primary antibiotics, but these most often represent colonization of the respiratory tract rather then superinfection. It is only when such organisms are associated with signs and symptoms of new infection that additional antibiotic treatment should be given.

FUNGAL INFECTION

Still uncommon in general practice, fungal infections may occur in patients with underlying serious illness or in specific geographic areas. In the latter case, many of the infections are self-limited and of little importance, but they may occasionally be sufficiently progressive or life threatening as to require treatment. Amphotericin B is the agent generally used for such infections, but it must be given intravenously and is quite toxic. Treatment is usually given with increasing dosage to the point of either sufficient therapy or major adverse effects, which include hypersensitivity reactions, hypokalemia, anemia and, most importantly, progressive abnormality of renal function.

Histoplasmosis

Histoplasmosis, prevalent in North American river valleys, is a relatively common but generally unimportant infection that occurs after inhalation of mycelia from contaminated soil. This leads to a flu-like illness that is generally self-limiting, but it may be associated with hilar adenopathy or pulmonary infiltrates. Residual calcifications in the lung may be a diagnostic concern but are of little consequence. Disseminated infection, which may occur in very young or very old patients or in patients with underlying illness, is associated with systemic symptoms, hepatosplenomegaly, lymphoadenopathy, anemia, and a variety of other manifestations, including diffuse pulmonary lesions. The infected organ may have to be biopsied so that the diagnosis can be made. Treatment, which is imperative, should be instituted with amphotericin. Chronic pulmonary histoplasmosis may simulate pulmonary tuberculosis, but the organisms should be present in the sputum.

Coccidiomycosis

Coccidiomycosis occurs in the southwestern United States and also is most commonly associated with a subclinical infection resulting from inhalation of the spores. The mild flu-like illness is generally self-limited, with or without pulmonary infiltrates. The disease may be associated with erythema nodosum and may resemble sarcoidosis. Disseminated disease is associated with involvement of multiple organ systems and is best evaluated by serial complement fixation studies, which are the guide to therapy with amphoteri-cin B.

Cryptococcosis

Unlike the organisms responsible for histoplasmosis and coccidiomycosis, Cryptococcus neoformans is widely distributed in the soil and may occur anywhere in the United States. Often associated with meningitis, the cryptococcus may produce a progressive disease of the lung suggesting granulomatosis or tuberculosis.

Aspergillosis

Aspergillus fumigatus is also widely distributed in nature and is frequently found in the airways of patients with asthma or with a characteristic form of pronounced, central bronchiectasis. Another important form of aspergillosis is colonization of a cavity, such as a healed tuberculous or abscess cavity. Colonization begins as thickening of the cavity wall, often misinterpreted as pleural thickening, and grows to a round density within the cavity. It may move on a change in position. These fungus balls may cause cough and even severe hemorrhage that occasionally requires surgical resection. The asper-gillus may also invade pulmonary tissue, with necrotizing pneumonia and dissemination to other organs, particularly in patients with immune defi-ciency, and may require treatment with amphotericin B.

Nocardiosis

Nocardia is also widely distributed in nature and may cause puzzling infection, manifest either as necrotizing pneumonia or occasionally as a persistent mass lesion, which can be misinterpreted as carcinoma of the lung. Lung biopsy may be necessary for diagnosis. Treatment with sul-fadiazine is often effective, but disseminated infection carries a very high mortality.

Pneumocystosis

Pneumocystis carinii is now recognized as a common cause of rapidly progressive pneumonia in the severely compromised host and such patients should either receive definitive diagnosis by transbronchial or needle or open biopsy of the lung or their infection should be treated by a very broad spectrum of antibiotics, including trimethoprim.

LUNG ABSCESS

Pathogenesis

Lung abscess most commonly results from aspiration of a large dose of oral bacteria after a period of unconsciousness. The organisms grow within the alveoli, producing necrosis of tissue and the ultimate formation of an abscess. This is most likely to occur in individuals with impaired mucociliary clearance, as from excessive ingestion of alcohol, or after a period of anesthesia. Less commonly, the abscess may occur distal to occlusion of a bronchus by a foreign body.

Lung abscess may also be the direct result of necrotizing pneumonia, as from a staphylococcal or klebsiella infection. Under these circumstances, the illness is more acute, with fever, chills, and cough, and usually leads to necrosis of the lung tissue and evident abscess formation on the roentgenogram in a few days. There have been reports of more indolent pulmonary infection with these organisms, leading to lung abscess more slowly.

Lung abscess is also a common finding in patients with bronchogenic carcinoma. A tumor may obstruct the bronchus, leading to poor drainage and infection of the distal lung, with ultimate breakdown and abscess formation. Such an abscess is in no way different from the lesion occurring after aspiration. In addition, a large tumor may outgrow its blood supply, with central necrosis and, ultimately, evacuation of central contents with abscess formation. A necrotizing tumor is more apt to have a thick, irregular wall, but the radiographic features are, again, not distinctive.

Finally, a lung cyst or bulla may become infected, and the clinical features and x-ray appearance are little different from a primary lung abscess.

Clinical Features

In most patients with aspiration lung abscess there is a relatively long history of cough and fever. Patients usually expectorate considerable quantities of purulent material, which is often foul smelling, and blood streaking or actual hemoptysis is common. Radiographic examination is essential for definition of the lesion, and it usually reveals an abscess cavity with an air fluid level. Clubbing of the fingers is not uncommon. One should obtain a careful history of the events leading up to the illness in order to make a diagnosis of aspiration lung abscess. There should have been a period of unconsciousness, often associated with the ingestion of excessive amounts of alcohol, or of fever, suggestive of pneumonia following surgery under general anesthesia. Almost all patients with pyogenic abscess have very poor oral hygiene and the absence of teeth suggests the likelihood of another etiological agent, such as a carcinoma of the lung leading to obstructive pneumonitis with abscess formation. Radiographic examination should include tomography for evaluation of the airway proximal to the abscess.

All patients with lung abscess do not require diagnostic bronchoscopy. If there is any suggestion of aspiration of a foreign body, the procedure must be performed so that this can be removed. In addition, if the clinical setting is not one in which abscess should develop, bronchoscopy is indicated for exclusion of a primary bronchogenic carcinoma, particularly in a heavy smoker or a patient with good oral hygiene. Otherwise, bronchoscopy may be delayed until treatment has been started and only performed if the expected resolution fails to occur.

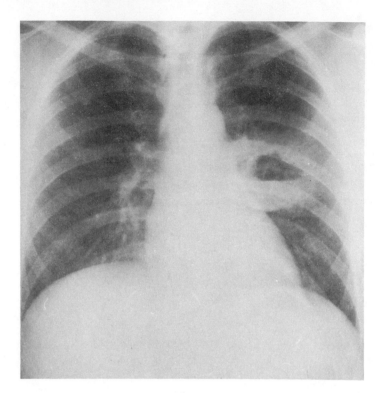

Figure 4–3 Lung abscess cavity containing air-fluid level in left mid lung field.

Treatment and Course

Although a variety of anaerobic organisms may well be responsible for some of the infection, it is now clear that the vast majority of patients will respond very well to moderate doses of penicillin, no more than 1.2 million units per day. If the therapeutic response is inadequate, one must be particularly careful in performing anaerobic cultures and searching for the causative organisms, which may be resistant to these or even higher doses of penicillin. Under those circumstances, the penicillin can be increased to as much as 20 million units per day or other agents such as clindamycin can be added. However, it must be emphasized that, regardless of the bacteriology of expectorated sputum or nasotracheal aspirates, almost all patients will respond to lower doses of penicillin. With treatment, one can expect gradual decrease of fever to normal levels within two weeks but a very much slower decrease in the size of the cavity. Initially, there should be reduction of the inflammatory reaction around the cavity, but closure cannot be expected for several weeks or months. In some patients the cavity never closes completely, but a thin-walled, noninfected air space remains permanently in the lung.

The other important aspect of therapy is the establishment of good drainage from the abscess cavity. It is essential that patients employ postural drainage designed to evacuate abscess contents so that they can cough up the infected material rather than have it aspirated into other parts of the lung. There are a number of case reports of individuals in whom the contents of the abscess cavity spontaneously drained into other parts of the lung, leading to massive pneumonia and adult respiratory distress syndrome. The cooperative patient can easily perform postural drainage with cough three or four times a day so as to prevent this complication. Patients should sleep in a position with the abscess cavity down so that, during sleep, there will not be excessive drainage into adjacent lung.

If postural drainage fails, it may be necessary to attempt other measures. Bronchoscopy has been performed successfully, but this must be done under local anesthesia so as not to have massive aspiration follow the bronchoscopy, with resultant flooding of normal lung. Most critical is the provision of postural drainage following the bronchoscopy. Alternatively, in very ill or badly obtunded patients, it has been possible to drain filled abscess cavities by percutaneous insertion of a chest tube. In most instances, within two or three weeks after development of the abscess the associated pleurisy provides a firm symphysis between visceral and a parietal pleura, so that a catheter can be inserted into the abscess without the danger of empyema or pneumothorax. An alternative to this approach is direct resection, but most surgeons would prefer to establish drainage of the abscess before surgery. With appropriate antibiotic therapy and postural drainage, surgical resection is rarely required.

The leading indication for surgery today is major hemoptysis. Hemoptysis is common in lung abscess, and it is usually far more serious than the hemoptysis associated with other lung lesions. Because of the high mortality, many believe that a large hemorrhage in a patient with lung abscess is an indication for emergency resection. Others would be willing to continue medical therapy in an effort to control the hemorrhage before resorting to surgery, but the patient's blood should be typed and cross-matched and surgical consultations sought if major hemoptysis develops.

Additional Reading

Briggs DD Jr: Pulmonary Infections. Clin North Am 61:1163–1183, 1977.
Reeder GS, Gracey DR: Aspiration of Intrathoracic Abscess. JAMA 240:1156–1159, 1978.
Reichman LB, McDonald RJ: Practical Management and Control of Tuberculosis. Med Clin North Am 61:1185–1204, 1977.

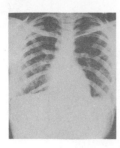

CHAPTER FIVE

DIFFUSE LUNG DISEASE

There are great many diseases that cause diffuse abnormality of the lung parenchyma. The lung interstitium, alveolar walls, or airspaces may become infiltrated with a wide variety of cells, fluid, or fibrous tissue, producing diffuse opacities on the x-ray film of the chest. The x-ray pattern may be predominantly alveolar, characterized by fluffy infiltrates enclosing patent bronchi (air bronchogram), or interstitial, which may be either nodular or linear. Unfortunately the patterns are often nonspecific and nondistinctive, so that one cannot make a diagnosis of the type of diffuse lung disease present from examination of the roentgenogram. In addition, the roentgenogram is a relatively insensitive indicator of the extent of the disease. Diffuse interstitial disease may even be present without apparent abnormality on the x-ray film.

These diseases are characterized by similar changes of pulmonary function, notably reduction of lung volumes because of encroachment of the disease process upon the airspaces and stiffening of the lung by inflammatory and fibrous tissue. Although all lung volumes are reduced, the vital capacity is affected as much as any and is a simple, reliable reflection of the severity of the process. In addition, the involvement of alveolar walls causes reduction of the diffusing capacity, which is another sensitive indicator of the extent of the disease. The disease may be acute, as in interstitial penumonia, or chronic, as in interstitial fibrosis, with a wide range in between. Very often the diagnosis is dependent upon obtaining a sample of lung tissue either by transbronchial biopsy or by an open-lung biopsy.

Diffuse interstitial disease of the lung can be produced by a number of infections. Acute pneumonia, as with influenza or mycoplasma, may produce an interstitial reaction, and chronic interstitial fibrosis is a result of other infections, such as tuberculosis. Diffuse miliary densities are characteristic of miliary tuberculosis and of some disseminated fungal infections. Diffuse interstitial involvement is also characteristic of pulmonary congestion, which is suggested by the presence of Kerly B lines and redistribution of the vascular pattern to the upper lobes. Chronic pulmonary congestion, particularly from mitral stenosis, causes diffuse interstitial fibrosis. Lymphangitic spread of carcinoma also produces diffuse interstitial infiltrates and restrictive lung disease (Fig. 5–1). This chapter will consider other diseases that cause primary diffuse interstitial disease of the lung.

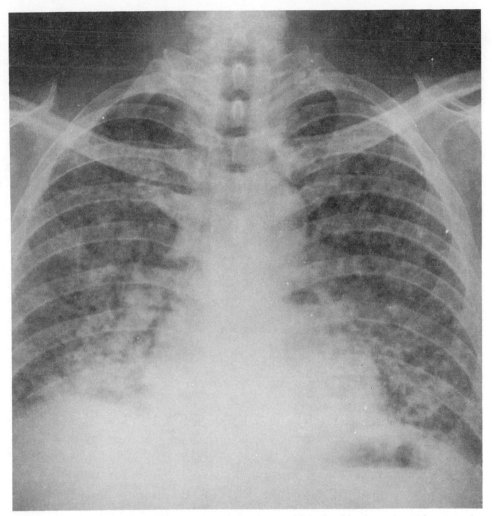

Figure 5–1 Diffuse interstitial disease of the lung which, in this case, turned out to be lymphangitic spread of carcinoma.

In some cases, as described later, there is specific therapy for the diffuse lung disease. In others, corticosteroids or immunosuppressants may produce substantial improvement. If in doubt, and if a specific cause has been excluded, it is reasonable to treat with 40 mg of prednisone for a month to see if improvement of vital capacity, which is usually evident within two weeks, occurs. If not, one may then embark upon a similar trial with azathioprine. Other therapy is supportive. Oxygen, even if given only at night, may prevent polycythemia, and portable oxygen may improve exercise tolerance and quality of life. Diuretics are useful in treating congestive heart failure.

SARCOIDOSIS

Pathogenesis

Sarcoidosis is a chronic, often benign disease characterized by the presence of noncaseating granuloma in various organs of the body. It is extremely common, more so than tuberculosis in many parts of the country, and it is world-wide in distribution. The etiology is unknown, but the sarcoid granuloma can be viewed as a battle ground between an indigestable antigen and the immune response to it. There is evidence that the initial reaction, the granuloma, represents migration and multiplication of macrophages in response to some unknown antigen, that these macrophages then become epithelioid cells or giant cells, leading to the formation of the characteristic, monotonously similar granuloma present in the involved organs.

It should be emphasized that these granulomas are not specific. Although characteristic of sarcoidosis, they can occur in a variety of other illnesses, including tuberculosis. Secretory products released by these macrophages may impair the function of T-lymphocytes, leading to the depression of cell-mediated immunity, which is characteristic of sarcoidosis. This, in turn, may be responsible for the excessive production of globulins by B-lymphocytes, accounting for the hyperglobulinemia, which is also common in the disease. The granulomatous inflammation is reflected in elevation of a number of serum enzymes, including lysozyme and angiotension-converting enzyme, which may represent markers of the extent and severity of illness. However, these assays have not yet proven to be specific for sarcoid or of great diagnostic value.

Sarcoid granulomas most commonly develop in the lung and hilar lymph nodes, suggesting that the antigen is initially inhaled. They may then be found in any part of the body, perhaps because of hematogenous spread of the antigen, but they are most prevalent and evident in the thorax. Sarcoidosis is usually associated with visible hilar adenopathy on the x-ray film of the chest, and most patients have evidence of abnormality of lung function resulting from the interstitial involvement with granuloma. The granulomas may ultimately disappear, or they may gradually become converted to fibrous tissue. The scarring of the lung resulting from interstitial fibrosis leads to the chronic, occasionally symptomatic restriction of lung function.

The immunologic abnormalities, particularly the cutaneous anergy, are useful diagnostic features of the illness, and a more specific test is provided by the intradermal injection of Kveim antigen, obtained from an extract of the spleen from a patient with sarcoidosis, which produces a characteristic granulomatous reaction. A positive Kveim test is thought to be highly specific for sarcoidosis and is almost always present, but unfortunately standardized antigen is not generally available for diagnostic use. The Kveim reaction may represent a miniature picture of the disease, coupling the etiological agent, the antigen, with the abnormal immune response.

Clinical Features

Sarcoidosis is most often manifest as asymptomatic, bilateral hilar lymphadenopathy (Fig. 5–2). It is frequently detected by x-ray screening of the populations such as military recruits. In the absence of systemic illness or pathology on physical examination and history, bilateral hilar adenopathy in an asymptomatic patient strongly suggests a diagnosis of sarcoidosis. Tuberculosis is rarely associated with a similar picture, primary infection causing unilateral hilar adenopathy, and the tuberculin test should be

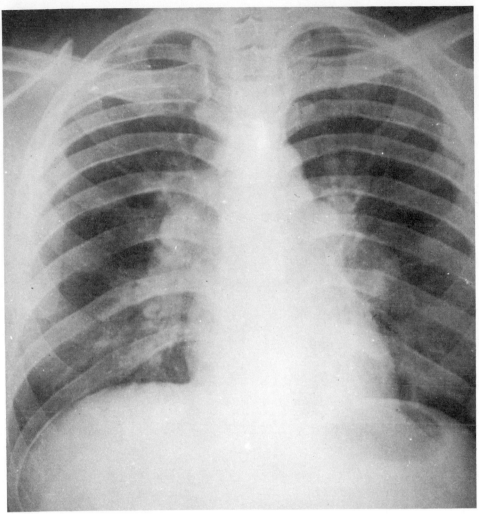

Figure 5–2 A young male with bilateral hilar adenopathy characteristic of sarcoidosis.

positive. Lymphoma, the other main diagnostic consideration, should be evident as lymphadenopathy elsewhere in the body and, generally, produces constitutional symptoms. Erythema nodosum occasionally is present at the onset of sarcoidosis. There are those who believe that asymptomatic hilar adenopathy, particularly if accompanied by erythema nodosum, is sufficient to make a diagnosis of sarcoidosis. Others would wish to obtain pathological material, by bronchial therapy or mediastinoscopy, in order to identify the granuloma and to exclude other conditions.

The lung is frequently involved, and abnormalities of lung function, particularly of the diffusing capacity, are often present, even in patients without evidence of abnormality on the x-ray film of the chest. In others, the x-ray reveals a varying degree of reticular nodular infiltration (Fig. 5–3) or, on occasion, large conglomerate lesions, occasionally resembling metastatic carcinoma, composed of the sarcoid granuloma (Fig. 5–4). Ultimately these

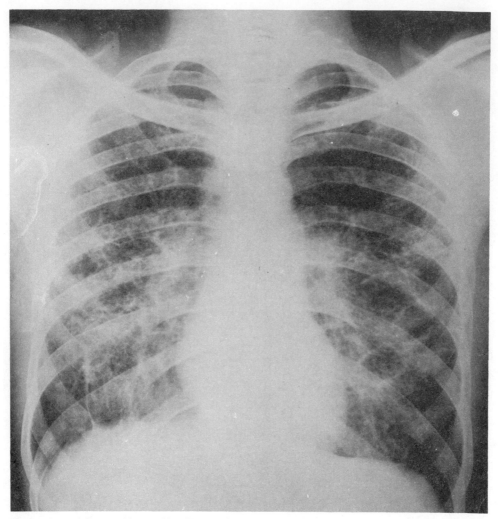

Figure 5–3 Advanced interstitial fibrosis from sarcoidosis with diffuse fibronodular scarring.

lesions generally regress, to be replaced by a variable degree of fibrous tissue. In some patients, the illness is heralded by the presence of systemic symptoms, including fever, and there may be evidence of involvement of almost any organ system. Granulomas are commonly present in the liver, resulting in abnormal liver function; there may be hematological abnormalities; and an enlarged spleen is occasionally present. One common feature of sarcoidosis is involvement of the eye, and a slit-lamp examination followed by biopsy of visible conjunctival lesions may reveal granulomas, which are sufficient to make a diagnosis. Hypercalcemia is another common finding; although its cause is not entirely clear, it may be sufficiently serious to require therapy with corticosteroids.

Although, as mentioned, there are sufficiently characteristic clinical syndromes to warrant a diagnosis of sarcoidosis without further study, in most instances the diagnosis requires the demonstration of a typical granuloma in some part of the body. Mediastinal and conjunctival granulomas

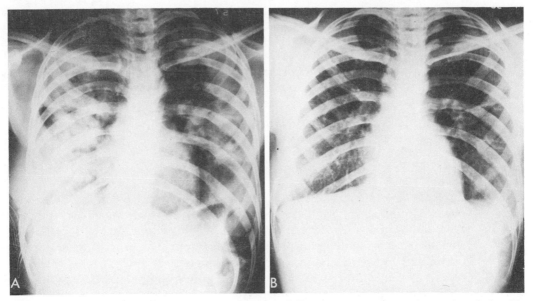

Figure 5-4 *(A)* Multiple infiltrates, suggestive of an inflammatory process or tumor, in a lady with severe dyspnea and marked impairment of pulmonary function (reduction of lung volumes and diffusing capacity). Lung biopsy revealed granuloma suggestive of sarcoidosis, and treatment with corticosteroids was associated with marked improvement of the roentgenogram *(B)*. There was, characteristically, increase of lung volumes and of diffusing capacity but not to normal.

are highly characteristic, but in many instances the simplest approach is to obtain tissue by bronchial and transbronchial biopsy through a fiberoptic bronchoscope. In some series, bronchoscopy reveals granuloma in close to 100 per cent of patients with sarcoidosis. It must be re-emphasized that granulomas are by no means specific for sarcoidosis but may represent a response to infection with tuberculosis or, even, a reaction to neoplastic tissue, as in lung cancer. In essence, the diagnosis of sarcoidosis is made when a patient with findings characteristic of the disease is found to have granulomas that cannot be explained by some other illness.

Figure 5-5 Serial measurements of vital capacity (VC) and of diffusing capacity (Dco) in a 26 year old lady with sarcoidosis. In most patients the extent of disease is evident within 1 to 2 years of onset and, as in this case, there is little further deterioration of pulmonary function over the ensuing years.

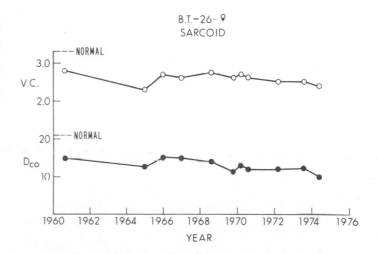

In the vast majority of cases sarcoidosis is a totally benign disease. Hilar adenopathy may slowly disappear or may be associated with or followed by the development of pulmonary infiltrates, which then generally improve or become attenuated as fibrous tissue replaces the granulomas. In almost all patients the disease will become fully established within a year or two of onset, and it is very uncommon for new pathology to develop after this time or for the granulomatous reaction to progress in an organ that has been involved from the beginning (Fig. 5–5).

Treatment

The only treatment available for sarcoidosis is corticosteroids, which apparently suppress the inflammatory reaction, improve organ function, and relieve symptoms. Corticosteroids are indicated for patients with symptoms, such as fever, or with serious organ involvement. The lung is the organ most commonly and seriously involved, and there is clear evidence that corticosteroids will cause improvement of reduced lung function. Obviously, patients with severe pulmonary insufficiency should receive corticosteroids, and many people believe that patients with even moderate impairment of lung function should also be treated. If improvement is induced, the dose of steroids should be reduced and continued at a level sufficient to maintain optimum pulmonary function (Fig. 5–6). This is best and most easily assessed by measurement of vital capacity. One approach is to give the patient 40 mg of prednisone per day; if the vital capacity is increased by more than 20 per cent after two weeks of treatment, the dose can gradually be reduced over a period of several months, following the vital capacity to be sure that it does not fall. It has been found that most patients who do experience improvement will relapse when corticosteroids are stopped, and therapy generally has to be maintained for at least two years and often much longer.

It is not clear whether or not patients with sarcoidosis are unusually

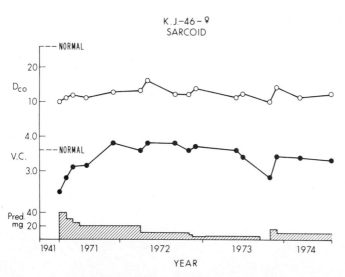

Figure 5–6 Serial pulmonary function studies in a 46 year old lady with sarcoidosis. Note the prompt improvement of vital capacity (VC) after institution of steroid therapy and the reversible deterioration that occurred when treatment was stopped three years later. It is common for the vital capacity to improve more than the diffusing capacity (Dco) perhaps because a decrease in the size of granuloma causes increase of lung volume without increasing the size of the pulmonary vascular bed available for diffusion.

susceptible to the development of tuberculosis. Probably they are not, but if a patient has had a previous infection, reflected in a positive tuberculin test in the past, or if a patient lives in an urban area that may be endemic for tuberculosis, it is probably wise to couple the administration of corticosteroids with prophylactic isoniazid, 300 mg per day.

Corticosteroids are also indicated for other serious manifestations of the disease. These include, particularly, uveitis, which may respond to local steroids, and significant hypercalcemia. Cardiac arrhythmias, or conduction disturbances on electrocardiography, suggest the presence of potentially serious myocardial involvement and are probably an indication for corticosteroid therapy.

Complications

Extensive involvement of the lung with pulmonary fibrosis may lead to such severe restrictive disease as to cause dynspnea and, ultimately, cor pulmonale. As in any kind of diffuse disease of the lung, therapy is largely supportive. The patients with chronic hypoxemia and resultant polycythemia will benefit from chronic oxygen therapy, and portable oxygen may make it possible for the disabled patient to experience a limited activity. Systemic venous congestion and edema, the result of pulmonary hypertension and cor pulmonale, is appropriately treated with diuretics, but digitalis is probably not indicated unless there is evidence of left ventricular failure.

It is known that sarcoid granulomas are frequently present in the airways of the lung, as well as in the interstitium, which is why bronchial biopsy is so often positive even in patients without evidence of airway obstruction. These granulomas may ultimately constrict airways, leading, by a check valve mechanism, to cavity formation in the lung. Such cavities are particularly susceptible to the development of infection with aspergillus, often evident at the onset by thickening of the cavity wall, which has the appearance of oblique thickening of the adjacent pleura but is actually due to fungal infection of the cavity itself. Later the movable density, partially surrounded by a crescent of air, becomes visible. These fungus balls are serious because they are often associated with hemoptysis, but they are not susceptible to treatment with antibiotics. In most instances, hemoptysis occurs in a patient with such extensive diffuse involvement of the lung that surgery is not possible, but if the involvement is less extensive resection may be indicated for severe, life-threatening bleeding or for recurring hemorrhages.

INTERSTITIAL PNEUMONITIS AND FIBROSIS

Usual Interstitial Pneumonia (UIP)

Chronic interstitial lung disease is frequently the result of a chronic interstitial reaction that ranges from inflammation to fibrosis (Fig. 5–7). The pathological changes are nonspecific and may result from a variety of known

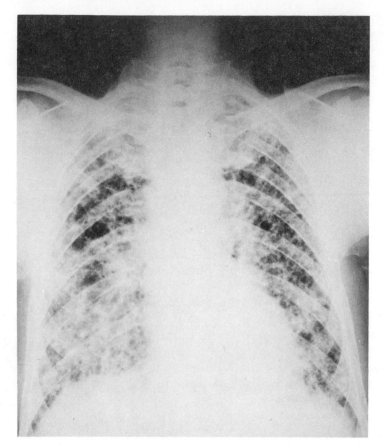

Figure 5–7 Extensive interstitial fibrosis of the lung.

agents, such as drugs and dusts, or as a component of systemic disease, as in scleredema. Usual interstitial pneumonia is the term now applied to patients in whom the interstitial reaction is of unknown cause. Other descriptive terms include idiopathic interstitial pneumonia, idiopathic interstitial fibrosis, and fibrosing alveolitis. The disease may be extremely rapid in onset and development and lead to death in a few weeks, as originally described in a group of patients by Hamman and Rich. More commonly, it is slowly progressive but frequently associated with crippling restrictive lung disease. The presence of immune complexes in the circulation suggests that, in many patients, UIP involves an abnormal immune response.

Patients with UIP frequently present with increasing shortness of breath, often associated with dry cough. Physical examination commonly reveals characteristic close-to-the-ear, cellophane, inspiratory crackles at the bases. An interstitial reaction is evident on roentgenogram, but the extent of the disease is far better reflected in reduction of lung volumes and of diffusing capacity. It is important to exclude known causes of the interstitial reaction by careful history of drug ingestion and occupational exposure. In most instances it is necessary to examine pulmonary tissues so as to exclude other specific diseases. In most centers this is first done by transbronchial biopsy through a fiberoptic bronchoscope and, if that is unsuccessful, by open-lung biopsy. In patients with clear evidence of extensive fibrosis, reflected in a honeycomb appearance on x-ray and a long duration of illness, the biopsy may be less important, since the likelihood of discovering a specific pathological lesion that is potentially reversible is so slim.

The course and the response to therapy depend upon the degree to which the inflammatory or fibrotic reaction predominates. An active inflammatory component is associated with a much better prognosis and with a much better response to corticosteroids. It is not necessary to obtain a lung biopsy to determine this, since in almost all cases a trial of steroid therapy, monitored by measurements of at least lung volumes, is indicated. The use of steroids will then be governed by the response, as in sarcoidosis. If steroids are unsuccessful, immunosuppressants may be tried.

Desquamative Interstitial Pneumonia (DIP)

One possibly unique pattern of interstitial reaction is associated with extensive desquamation of alveolar cells into the airspaces with less interstitial infiltrate than is present in UIP. DIP is apparently associated with a much better prognosis and a better response to corticosteroids, but whether or not it represents a different disease is not entirely clear.

Eosinophilic Granuloma

Pulmonary eosinophilic granuloma is characterized by proliferation of histiocytes in the interstitium of the lung with variable degrees of necrosis and fibrosis. In about 20 per cent of patients it is associated with lesions in the bone or with involvement of the posterior pituitary gland, causing diabetes insipidus. Cough and dyspnea are no different than in other forms of interstitial disease, though inspiratory crackles are far less common than in UIP. It is not generally associated with eosinophilia or abnormalities of bone marrow, but mild anemia is common. It is frequently associated with pneumothorax because of the development of small cystic spaces in the lung, visible as a honeycomb appearance on the roentgenogram in advanced stages. The course is very unpredictable, with occasional instances of spontaneous improvement or progressive worsening. In most cases, however, the disease remains relatively static and without progression over many years. No therapy, including corticosteroids, has been shown to be of benefit. Diagnosis can only be made with certainty by lung biopsy.

Intrapulmonary Hemorrhage

There are two different conditions associated with widespread alveolar hemorrhage.

Idiopathic Pulmonary Hemosiderosis

Idiopathic pulmonary hemosiderosis is a disease that most commonly involves children or young adults and is manifest as recurrent episodes of hemoptysis and iron deficiency anemia. The diffuse interstitial disease on the roentgenogram is distinctively alveolar in nature with fluffy infiltrates and an air bronchogram, and the lesions tend to occur episodically, with the development of a variable degree of pulmonary fibrosis. Massive and even fatal hemoptysis may occur. There have been reports of this rare disorder occurring in members of the same family, suggesting a genetic basis. Both corticosteroids and immunosuppressant drugs have been reported as being effective, but their role has not been clearly established. The course is usually one of remissions and exacerbations, with long periods of well-being between episodes of bleeding. Progressive impairment of pulmonary function may lead to restrictive lung disease, and fatal hemorrhage may occur at any time.

Goodpasture's Syndrome

Goodpasture's syndrome is a more virulent form of diffuse alveolar bleeding associated with glomerulonephritis and characterized by the presence of antibodies to the basement membrane of the glomeruli and, probably, of the lung. Attempts have been made to stem the progressive pulmonary hemorrhage by nephrectomy, by the use of immunosuppressive agents, and, more recently, by removing circulating antibodies by combining plasmapheresis with administration of prednisone and cyclophosphamide.

Serious, generally fatal, pulmonary hemorrhage has been associated with bleeding disorders and with systemic lupus erythematosus. It may also occur as a localized hematoma following direct injury to the chest, in which case it is generally of little consequence and gradually resolves.

Lymphoid Interstitial Pneumonia (LIP)

Another variant of chronic interstitial pneumonia is cellular infiltration with lymphocytes. This is a relatively benign disorder and is apt to respond favorably to corticosteroids. In some instances, it is a reflection of a systemic disorder, notably Sjögren's syndrome, and other patients reveal lymphadenopathy, hepatomegaly, and abnormalities of serum globulins. It is important to distinguish the condition, by careful study of biopsies, from the more serious pulmonary angiitis and granulomatosis to be discussed later. Lymphocytes may also infiltrate the lung in patients with lymphomas, and pneumonic clusters of lymphocytes may involve the lung without evidence of systemic disease, a disorder termed pseudolymphoma.

PULMONARY INFILTRATES WITH EOSINOPHILIA (PIE)

This is a group of disorders in which pulmonary infiltrates are accompanied by blood eosinophilia. They range from the benign, fleeting infiltrates of Loeffler's syndrome to a progressive systemic disorder associated with vasculitis (Table 5–1).

Table 5–1 Pulmonary Infiltrates with Eosinophilia (PIE)

Benign — Loeffler's syndrome
Tropical — microfiliaria
Bronchopulmonary aspergillosis
Eosinophilic pneumonia
Necrotizing vasculitis — Churg-Strauss syndrome
Drugs — sulfonamides

Loeffler's Syndrome

In Loeffler's syndrome the infiltrates are transient and self-limiting. The disease is mild and may be entirely asymptomatic. There is no need for therapy. In the tropics, eosinophilia and pulmonary infiltrates have been associated with a number of parasites, including microfilaria. In patients with asthma, pulmonary infiltrates may be related to infection with aspergillus. They usually respond to steroid therapy.

Eosinophilic Pneumonia

Eosinophilic pneumonia is a condition mainly affecting nonatopic people in which large areas of the lung are packed with eosinophils, often in a peripheral rather than central distribution, the opposite of pulmonary edema. This may be associated with asthma, and other symptoms include fever, sweats, weight loss, and progressive dyspnea. The response to treatment with corticosteroids is dramatic, large pneumonic infiltrates often disappearing rapidly, and it is important to establish the diagnosis by transbronchial biopsy so that therapy can be instituted promptly. Continuing treatment may be necessary to suppress recurrent symptoms but, to date, the prognosis has been excellent with such therapy.

Systemic Necrotizing Vasculitis

The most serious form of PIE is that associated with systemic necrotizing vasculitis. This syndrome, first reported by Churg and Strauss, occurs in atopic patients with asthma and is associated with fever and granulomatous vasculitis in other organs. It may evolve from a benign disorder identical to Loeffler's syndrome, or it may present with systemic symptoms from the onset. Churg-Strauss syndrome is very similar to periarteritis nodosa, but the diagnosis may be made by demonstrating necrotizing extravascular granuloma in the areas of involvement. Corticosteroids are used and, if not effective, should probably be followed by more potent agents such as cyclophosphamide or azathioprine.

There are many similarities between PIE, Wegener's granulomatosis, and periarteritis nodosa, but there are also, in the minds of pathologists, distinctive histological differences, and there are clinical differences. Wegener's is less likely to be associated with allergy, asthma, or eosinophilia, and there is striking involvement of kidneys and midline structures. Periarteritis affects larger vessels with infiltrates of polymorphonuclear leukocytes rather than eosinophils and is not associated with extravascular granuloma.

Nonetheless, these and other interstitial pneumonias and collagen vascular disease may have a common etiology and pathogenesis related to an abnormal immune response.

PULMONARY ANGIITIS AND GRANULOMATOSIS

Wegener's Granulomatosis

Wegener's granulomatosis is a systemic disease of adults characterized by necrotizing granuloma associated with vasculitis, particularly in the upper and lower respiratory tract and kidney. It is not generally associated with allergy or asthma and often presents with systemic symptoms. Pulmonary infiltrates are commonly present, as is sinusitis and abnormality of renal function. Upper airway involvement may be severe, with necrotizing, destructive lesions in the nasopharynx. Many other organs may be involved, and there have been reports of arthralgia, skin lesions, and neurological abnormalities. A limited form of the disease is restricted to the lung and has a much better prognosis than is present in patients with renal involvement. The latter generally progress rapidly to death, but it has now been shown that treatment with cyclophosphamide is extremely effective in inducing remission and preventing the otherwise high mortality. The diagnosis must be made by demonstrating characteristic lesions in areas of involvement and treatment should be instituted with cyclophosphamide (1–2 mg/kg) for two weeks. The dose should then be increased by increments of 25 mg until the renal disease is controlled or the clinical response is favorable or until the white blood count falls below 3,000 per cubic millimeter. It is generally felt that treatment should be continued for at least a year after resolution of disease activity, longer if symptoms or abnormalities persist.

Lymphomatoid Granulomatosis

This is a disease characterized by pulmonary infiltrates, often involving the bases of the lungs and associated with cough, fever, and dyspnea. The lesions consist of infiltration of lymphocytes associated with angiitis and clusters of infiltrating cells, which appear like granulomas. This is a serious, often progressive and fatal disease frequently associated with peripheral neuritis and skin lesions, which may lead to the diagnosis. There have been reports of a more benign form of illness limited to the lung. The diagnosis is made by lung biopsy, and in this disease it is important to obtain adequate tissue for careful study, since similarities to other types of more benign granuloma such as sarcoidosis or granulomatous infections or to lymphoma may be difficult to resolve with a small biopsy. There is evidence that treatment with cyclophosphamide is effective, and it is important to estab-lish the correct diagnosis so that this potentially dangerous treatment may be instituted promptly.

These diseases highlight the need to suspect serious disease requiring potentially toxic treatment in patients with pulmonary infiltrates. Fever and constitutional symptoms, evidence of extrapulmonary involvement, and an x-ray appearance of nonuniform, nodular as well as interstitial involvement all suggest the presence of such disease and the need for lung biopsy.

Collagen Vascular Disease

A number of variants of collagen vascular disease can produce radiographic, functional, and histological abnormalities in the lung similar both to interstitial pneumonia and to angiitis and granulomatosis. Scleroderma commonly involves the lungs, often only manifest as a reduction of the diffusing capacity but frequently associated with bilateral interstitial infiltrates. Lupus erythematosus may be accompanied by pulmonary infiltrates, but they are far less common than pleural effusion, which is a frequent manifestation of the disease. Rheumatoid arthritis may be associated with an increased incidence of diffuse interstitial fibrosis, and patients with UIP not infrequently have serological evidence of rheumatoid disease. Patients with rheumatoid arthritis respond to agents such as silica with a more pronounced inflammatory reaction in the lung (Kaplan's syndrome) than normals. Rheumatoid disease is also commonly associated with pleural effusions and with nodular lesions in the lung. Periarteritis nodosa may involve the lung and resemble PIE with vasculitis, but some of the differences were described previously. Sjögren's syndrome commonly involves the lung and has also been reported in association with lymphoid interstitial pneumonia.

HYPERSENSITIVITY PNEUMONITIS

Hypersensitivity pneumonitis, or extrinsic allergic alveolitis, results from the inhalation of organic antigens in susceptible individuals. Initially described as "farmer's lung," it occurred after inhalation of moldy hay contaminated by fungal organisms. Subsequently, a wide variety of occupations, hobbies, and living conditions have been associated with this reaction. Pigeon fanciers, detergent workers, mushroom pickers, cheese workers, and a great many other individuals have been described with the syndrome, and it has also been reported after inhalation of air contaminated by thermophilic actinomycetes growing in home air conditioners. Maple bark, wood pulp, cork dust, coffee beans, redwood sawdust, and a host of other materials, most of which are contaminated by fungi but some of which may be the antigen themselves, have been found to cause this syndrome. Clearly a careful history of occupational exposure, recent change of living quarters or air conditioning equipment, or even the use of drugs, notably intranasal vasopressin, is very important in making the diagnosis.

Symptoms characteristically occur 3 to 6 hours after inhalation of the offending agent and may include fever, malaise, arthralgias, dyspnea, cough, and chest discomfort. They probably represent a Type 3 allergic response from the reaction of the antigen with circulating precipitating antibodies. These symptoms may be preceded by asthma immediately after inhalation challenge, presumably a Type 1 allergic response of IgE antibodies. Inspiratory crackles are generally heard in the chest and the roentgenogram reveals a diffuse fibronodular reaction or fluffy alveolar infiltrates, which may persist for several days after exposure. Leukocytosis is generally present. There is generally reduction of lung volumes and of diffusing capacity, and occasionally airway obstruction is present. The symptoms usually subside within hours to days.

The condition should be suspected in a patient with recurrent illness of this sort and a source of exposure revealed by a careful history. Precipitating antibodies to thermophilic actinomycetes may be present in the blood, but their presence does not necessarily indicate the illness, since they are frequently present in exposed individuals who do not suffer the allergic response. The absence of precipitins is useful in excluding the diagnosis.

Treatment is avoidance of exposure. Severe symptoms respond promptly to the administration of corticosteroids. If exposure continues and illness recurs, it is likely to lead to chronic interstitial and obstructive disease of the lung because of involvement both of the interstitium and of airways. If this is allowed to happen, irreversible changes are apt to occur, although therapy with corticosteroids may be of some value, as in other types of interstitial lung disease or chronic obstructive disease. Pulmonary function studies become very helpful in assessing efficacy and adjusting the dosage of corticosteroids.

PNEUMOCONIOSIS

There are a number of effective mechanisms for protecting the lung from the damage threatened by continued inhalation of air contaminated by a variety of dusts and other substances, some of which have been discussed in previous chapters. The sticky lining of the airways traps large particles that are inhaled, and they are effectively swept up the mucociliary escalator to be swallowed or expectorated. Smaller particles, and these are the ones capable of causing damage, may be ingested by alveolar macrophages and subsequently cleared by lymphatics or the mucociliary mechanism. A large dose of an agent may overwhelm these mechanisms. Individuals with defective macrophage function from underlying illness or acute viral infection or individuals in whom the mucociliary mechanism has been damaged by cigarette smoke or chronic airway disease are more at risk than others.

Pneumoconiosis is the result of inhalation of small particles, generally less than 5 mcg in diameter, which cannot be effectively cleansed by these mechanisms. The degree of inflammation and ultimate fibrosis are dependent upon the nature of the dust, the intensity of the exposure, and the host reaction.

Silicosis

Silicosis results from the inhalation of small particles of free silicon dioxide and is generally the result of prolonged occupational exposure. The details of the history are very important in making the diagnosis. The principal industries associated with silicosis are mining, stone cutting, glass manufacture, and foundry work, but there are many others and the details of the occupation must be carefully described. Months to years of exposure may be necessary before the reaction occurs. It usually starts as small nodular lesions throughout the lungs, which may enlarge, coalesce, and cause large aggregates. In addition, the hilar lymph nodes may become enlarged and calcified, with a characteristic "eggshell" appearance. The extent of fibrosis in the lungs is best reflected in measurements of pulmonary function, and extensive fibrosis results in severe restrictive lung disease with, ultimately, respiratory failure and chronic hypoxia.

The diagnosis is made from the association of characteristic radiographic findings with a history of adequate exposure to silica. There is no specific therapy, but silicosis is frequently complicated by tuberculosis, and there are some who feel that the development of conglomerate disease with cavitation is always the result of mycobacterial infection. For that reason, patients with silicosis with a positive tuberculin test should receive a year of therapy with isoniazid, and patients with cavitary disease must be evaluated and treated as if they had active tuberculosis. This means institution of at least two active chemotherapeutic agents pending confirmation by culture.

Asbestosis

Asbestos is widely used in a number of industries, particularly among shipworkers, insulators, and individuals who work with brake linings and asbestos shingles. It has now been shown that very little exposure may lead to inhalation of the asbestos fiber. Particularly disconcerting is the knowledge that individuals who have merely worked in shipyards, even if not directly exposed to asbestos, are apt to have asbestos bodies in their lungs and to be at high risk for the development of lung cancer. Indeed, the families of asbestos workers, or people living near the plants, have been shown to be at risk. The most serious consequence of asbestosis is the development of lung cancer, particularly among cigarette smokers, and this may develop without previous lesions on x-ray. Exposed smokers are said to have a 100-fold risk of lung cancer. There is also an increased incidence of cancer of the abdominal organs and of mesothelioma of pleura and peritoneum. Pleural reactions with pleural effusions are very common in this type of pneumoconiosis, and a characteristic late lesion is the calcified pleural plaque at the base of the lung. Heavy exposure may lead to a chronic inflammatory reaction with diffuse interstitial fibrosis with disabling restrictive lung disease.

Asbestosis has become a major occupational hazard in the United States, and considerable attention is being devoted to preventing the exposure, which may not result in disease until 20 or 30 years later.

Berylliosis

Inhalation of even very small amounts of beryllium may lead to an extensive granulomatous lesion, presenting either as an acute pneumonitis or, later, as chronic pulmonary fibrosis. Acute exposure is associated with cough, chest pain, and dyspnea, which may slowly resolve only to be followed ultimately by the development of chronic interstitial fibrosis. The histological and clinical features are very similar to sarcoidosis, but beryllium may be identified in lung tissue by physical methods. Although berylliosis used to occur in workers making fluorescent light bulbs or, even, after exposure to a broken bulb, beryllium is no longer used in this process and is restricted to very limited areas such as aerospace research and nuclear reactors.

There is some evidence that a hypersensitivity reaction is involved in the reaction to beryllium and for that reason patients with progressive deterioration of lung function should be given corticosteroids, the effect to be evaluated as it is in sarcoidosis.

Coal Miner's Pneumoconiosis

Individuals who have worked as cutters in mines for many years have a very high instance of pneumoconiosis, in addition to silicosis, which is apparently the result of carbon pigments deposited in the lung. This starts as a finely reticular nodulation which, with repeated exposure, progresses to increasing fibrosis and, because of involvement of the airways, obstructive lung disease. Miners with rheumatoid arthritis may develop large nodules in the lung, which occasionally cavitate (Kaplan's syndrome). The propensity to coal worker's pneumoconiosis is greatly enhanced by cigarette smoking, and there are some who believe that the obstructive lesion is primarily the result of cigarette smoke rather than carbon.

Other Dusts

Some other dusts, such as talc, may also produce a progressive interstitial lung disease with significant impairment of lung function. Others, such as barium, tin, and iron produce a widely dispersed nodular reaction on x-ray that is not associated with significant limitation of lung function or of symptoms. Cadmium has caused an acute chemical pneumonitis, leading to the development of chronic obstructive pulmonary disease and emphysema.

DRUG REACTIONS

Just as the lung bears the brunt of assault by noxious agents in the inspired air, so too it is exposed to materials present in the circulation. All the blood flows through the lung, and it is now known that there are a number of important ways in which the pulmonary capillaries can identify and alter circulating material. It is not surprising that some potentially toxic agents can be concentrated in the lung and cause pulmonary injury. There is great variation in the type of adverse effect that can be produced, and some of these will be considered here. It should be emphasized that as new agents are introduced, and as we learn more about drugs that have already been in use, more and more pulmonary toxic effects will become apparent, both of the types to be discussed below and probably of forms not yet recognized.

Interstitial Pneumonitis

It is now known that a great many agents can produce interstitial lung disease, ranging from the early changes of edema and inflammation to chronic interstitial fibrosis. The most serious reactions are produced by some of the powerful agents used in the chemotherapy of cancer. Busulfan produces pulmonary fibrosis, which may not become apparent for many years after a course of therapy. Bleomycin, which is concentrated in the lung, also may produce a delayed reaction, but there is usually evidence of diffuse lung disease within six months of initiating therapy. Cyclophosphamide produces a similar reaction. Methotrexate, an antimetabolite, appears to produce a more reversible form of diffuse lung disease associated with eosinophilia in many patients, suggesting a hypersensitivity reaction. Toxicity may occur within 12 days of treatment but, again, may not be evidence for several years. There is no relationship to dosage, and of these drug reactions this is the only one that has responded to steroid therapy.

As with other types of interstitial pneumonitis, patients complain of cough, sometimes associated with fever and dyspnea. The roentgenogram reveals interstitial and alveolar infiltrates. Pulmonary function studies, which show restriction, are the most sensitive indicators of the extent of the illness. It is probably wise to monitor ventilatory function in patients treated with these agents, but the late appearance of the pulmonary reaction may preclude detection early enough to stop treatment in time to prevent injury. A lung biopsy is generally necessary to exclude progression of the underlying disease, such as angiitis or tumor, and complicating infection. Characteristic findings are large numbers of atypical Type II cells within the alveoli.

Radiation

Radiation produces interstitial pneumonitis, which, in the acute form, is associated with progressive pulmonary infiltrates within a few weeks of the onset of treatment. X-ray film of the chest may reveal a characteristic distribution, which does not follow lobar boundaries but does conform to the area of the lung that was radiated. The chronic form may appear 6 to 18 months after radiation has been started. The acute reaction is not dose related, and it may represent a hypersensitivity reaction; however, chronic interstitial lung disease is clearly dose related and is inevitable, to some degree, in patients who have received more than 6,000 rads. Pre-existent pulmonary disease does not appear to predispose to radiation injury, and there is no evidence that corticosteroids have a beneficial effect on it, but patients on steroid therapy may develop the pulmonary reaction to radiation if the steroids are discontinued. For this reason it is wise not to give radiation therapy to the lung in patients taking corticosteroids or, if the steroids are necessary, to continue to give them for six months after radiotherapy has been completed and, then, to taper the dose gradually.

Nitrofurantoin

Nitrofurantoin has been associated with an acute pulmonary reaction characterized by fever, dyspnea, cough, and diffuse alveolitis associated with pleural effusion not unlike pulmonary edema and occurring within a few hours to days after treatment. It is associated with eosinophilia and may lead to diffuse interstitial fibrosis. There is also a form of chronic disease associated with treatment with this antibiotic; it is characterized by episodic fever, progressive dyspnea and diffuse interstitial fibrosis, particularly at the bases. Corticosteroids have led to rapid improvement in some patients.

Cyclophosphamide

Cyclophosphamide, an alkylating agent used for the treatment of angiitis and granulomatosis, has also resulted in interstitial pneumonitis, generally slowly developing and occurring many months after onset of therapy. In a patient with a disease such as Wegener's granulomatosis on treatment with cyclophosphamide, a new pulmonary infiltrate may be the result of the drug, of progress of the underlying disease, or of superimposed infection. Lung biopsy may be needed to provide a definitive diagnosis, and it may be necessary to stop the therapy in order to learn whether or not the pulmonary reaction is drug related.

Oxygen

It is now known that high concentrations of oxygen, perhaps as little as 40 per cent over a long period of time, are associated with diffuse pneumonitis, which may ultimately progress to pulmonary fibrosis. It is for this reason that hypoxemic patients are treated with as little oxygen as necessary to maintain reasonably normal arterial blood oxygen tension. It is often very difficult to know whether oxygen or the underlying lung disease is responsible for the diffuse lung damage. In high concentrations, oxygen is associated with acute tracheobronchitis, manifest as substernal discomfort associated with cough. In addition to causing structural changes in the lungs, 100 per cent oxygen predisposes to atelectasis because the air in the oxygen-filled alveolus is rapidly absorbed following obstruction of a bronchus, as from excessive secretions.

Heavy Metals

Heavy metals may cause pulmonary fibrosis, and there have been reports of diffuse interstitial disease resulting from gold.

Respiratory Paralysis

The polymyxins and aminoglycosides have been reported to cause neuromuscular blockade, beginning between 1 and 24 hours after injection and lasting up to 3 days. Respiratory paralysis may be associated with evidence of myasthenia, such as diplopia, dysphagia, and ptosis. Respiratory depression is more apt to occur in patients with pre-existing neuromuscular disease, particularly myasthenia gravis.

Nosocomial Infections

Patients being treated with corticosteroids or an immunosuppressant, particularly after renal transplantation, are very much at risk of infection from organisms that are harmless to the normal host. *Pneumocystis carinii*, for which there is now specific antimicrobial therapy, is a notorious example of this, and a number of other fungi as well as bacteria and viruses can seriously infect the compromised host. For this reason, when a patient on such therapy develops fever and cough, even if the pulmonary infiltration is minimal, it is important to institute immediate hospitalization and either cover with very broad-spectrum antimicrobial therapy or proceed immediately to transbronchial or open-lung biopsy.

Pulmonary Infiltration with Eosinophilia (PIE)

A number of drugs, including sulfonamides and penicillin, have been associated with this syndrome. Lupus syndromes, with pleural effusions and pneumonic infiltrates, have been associated with a variety of drugs, particularly procainamide hydrochloride (Pronestyl). A similar reaction may occur with isoniazid, hydralazine, and phenytoin (Dilantin).

Pulmonary Edema

A number of reports have implicted various drugs in the development of acute pulmonary edema, probably because of diffuse capillary injury. This has been most commonly and convincingly associated with heroin overdose, the pulmonary edema occurring some hours after the intravenous injection of heroin and generally associated with profound respiratory depression. Prompt supportive therapy with naloxone and mechanical ventilation with intubation if necessary generally lead to complete resolution within a few days. It is not clear whether the pulmonary edema results from a toxic action of heroin on pulmonary capillaries or from hypoxia secondary to respiratory depression. A similar reaction may follow an overdose of methadone or the use of excessive amounts of sedatives, such as ethchlorvynol (Placidyl). It may be that the pulmonary edema is similar to the reaction that occasionally occurs at high altitudes and is clearly the result of hypoxia. It is also known that drug addicts are likely to have evidence of diffuse lung damage, reflected in reduction of diffusing capacity and perfusion defects on lung scan, variously interpreted as pulmonary emphysema or restriction of the pulmonary vascular bed secondary to granulomatosis.

PULMONARY ALVEOLAR PROTEINOSIS

Pulmonary alveolar proteinosis is a relatively new disorder characterized by the presence of large amounts of a lipoprotein material in the alveoli with very little tissue reaction. The cause is unknown, but it seems likely that the

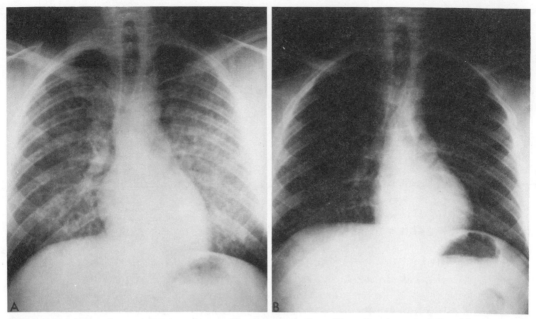

Figure 5–8 Extensive pulmonary edema with normal cardiac silhouette characteristic of heroin over-dose *(A)*. Two days later the roentgenogram was normal. (Reproduced from Williams, M. Henry: Pulmonary complications of drug abuse. *In* Fishman A. P. (ed.): Pulmonary Disease and Disorder. New York, McGraw-Hill, 1980, p. 1066).

substance within the alveoli is the normal phospholipid surfactant, which is imperfectly cleared from the alveolar spaces. Cough and dyspnea are common complaints and symptoms may progress, but the course is extremely variable, ranging from spontaneous remission to progressive pulmonary insufficiency and death. This form of diffuse lung disease is characteristically associated with an increased right-to-left shunt because blood continues to perfuse the capillaries of the unventilated alveoli. It has also been found that there are increases of lactic acid dehydrogenase (LDH) in the blood of patients with this disease. Although the radiographic finding of diffuse alveolar infiltrates may be suggestive, it is impossible to make a specific diagnosis from the x-ray, and other patterns may be present. This disorder is particularly likely in a patient with diffuse interstitial lung disease associated with right-to-left shunting and increased serum LDH. Since the hypoxemia is the result of a shunt, oxygen therapy is of little value, and it is essential to make the diagnosis promptly by lung biopsy in order to institute specific therapy.

Treatment has been successful both by aerosol therapy with proteolytic enzymes and by lung lavage. The latter has been the most consistently successful approach, but it involves general anesthesia and special skill and facilities. Lavage is followed by retrieval of large amounts of lipoprotein from the lungs, associated with radiographic, physiological, and symptomatic improvement, but it may have to be repeated intermittently for exacerbations of the disease. Corticosteroids are without value in this condition and may predispose to serious pulmonary infections, which account for many of the deaths.

Additional Reading

Carrington CB, Gaensler EA, et al: Natural history and treated course. N Engl J Med 298:801–809, 1978.

Chumbley LC, Harrison EG, DeReMae RA: Allergic granulomatosis and angiitis (Churg-Strauss Syndrome). Mayo Clinic Proc 52:477–484, 1977.

Colp C: Sarcoidosis: course and treatment. Med Clin North Am 61:1267–1278, 1977.

Liebow AA: Pulmonary angiitis and granulomatosis. Am Rev Resp Dis 108:1, 1973.

Lipmann M: Pulmonary reactions to drug. Med Clin North Am 61:1353–1368, 1977.

Pearson DJ, Rosenow EL: Chronic eosinophilic pneumonia (Carrington's). Mayo Clinic Proc 53:73, 1978.

Shanies H: Noncardiogenic pulmonary edema. Med Clin North Am 61:1319–1338, 1977.

Strimlan CV, Rosenow EC 3rd, Weiland LH, et al: Lymphocytic interstitial pneumonitis. Review of 13 cases. Ann Inter Med 88:616–621, 1978.

Zeck RT, Cugell BW: Diffuse infiltration lung disease. Med Clin North Am 61:1251–1266, 1977.

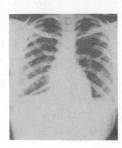

CHAPTER SIX

LUNG CANCER

Relatively rare 40 years ago, lung cancer has become the leading cause of death in men from malignant disease in the United States. In this country, as in others, the explosive increase of lung cancer has closely paralleled, after many years, an increase in cigarette smoking. Indeed, it is now occurring with increasing frequency among women who began smoking in greater numbers in the 1940's. There are many other known carcinogenic inhalants, including asbestos, nickel, and uranium. Men who worked in shipyards during World War II, and even the members of their family who came in contact with their dusty clothing, are at great risk of developing lung cancer from exposure to asbestos. Neoplastic transformation is also associated with previous pulmonary pathology and is likely to develop in damaged areas of the lung, such as scars.

The most common form of lung cancer is squamous cell carcinoma, which originates in bronchi and spreads to hilar lymph nodes and, then, distant sites of the body. Adenocarcinomas are apt to arise at more distal sites in the lung, particularly in association with scars. The prognosis and results of surgical treatment are not closely related to the type of carcinoma, although the highly anaplastic oat cell carcinoma is so prone to metastasize before it is clinically evident that, with the exception of very small lesions, it is no longer considered a surgical condition. Other tumors, such as alveolar cell carcinoma and papillary tumors, have unique clinical features, which will be discussed in this chapter. In general, lung tumors grow so slowly and produce so few symptoms that they tend to metastasize and become incurable before they can be detected and treated successfully. The overall mortality from this disease is about 90 per cent, and it is little better if semiannual x-ray examinations are performed in persons at risk. By the time the tumor is apparent on the x-ray film, it has generally metastasized. Nonetheless, there are tumors that can be detected early enough to be cured, and it is very important for the physician to be mindful of the various ways in which they can present and to have an understanding of the surgical and other therapeutic approaches that are available for treatment. The only real hope, however, for controlling this usually fatal illness is the abolition of cigarette smoking.

Figure 6–1 Solitary nodule in the upper half of the lung in an asymptomatic man proved to be a squamous cell carcinoma. Although the diagnosis of such a lesion may be established by transbronchial biopsy, in many cases, particularly in smaller lesions, the nature of the abnormality can only be ascertained by surgical resection. (Reproduced with permission from Fraser, RG, and Paré, JAP: Diagnosis of Diseases of the Chest. 2nd edition. Philadelphia, W. B. Saunders Company, 1979, p. 1050.)

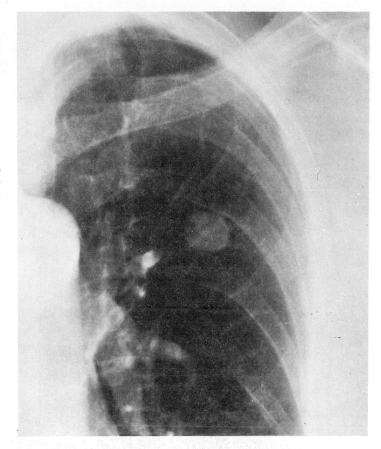

CLINICAL PRESENTATIONS

Coin Lesions

Of all the forms of lung cancer, the small, solid lesion detected on x-ray examination of the asymptomatic patient is the type that is most likely to be cured by surgical resection (Fig. 6–1). Although many of these lesions have already spread to distant sites at the time of detection, enough of them are curable to make it extremely important to pay attention to any such radiographic finding. There are a number of factors that make a coin lesion so likely to be cancer as to warrant prompt resection. These include a history of cigarette smoking, age, and the absence of other granulomatus disease on the x-ray.

There are no truly distinctive features in the x-ray appearance of the lesion, but tomographic study is important to exclude calcification, which is almost always associated with a benign granuloma, and the presence of other lesions. It is particularly important to obtain previous x-rays in an effort to learn whether or not the lesion has been present in the past. If it has not changed over a period of years, careful observation is appropriate. Sputum specimens may be obtained, if necessary by artificial induction, to search for malignant cells. Transbronchial biopsy may be attempted in order to obtain a diagnosis, but this is usually nonrevealing. If the biopsy does reveal tumor, surgery will certainly be done, but one cannot rely on nonspecific findings such as fibrosis and granuloma, both of which may be associated with tumors, to be certain that the lesion is benign. If any question remains, the lesion should be removed.

In the final analysis, the physician and patient together must often make a judgment whether to perform surgery for what may be a benign lesion or to observe serial x-ray films to detect increasing size and run the risk of operating too late.

Mass Lesions

There is a wide variety of presentations of patients with larger tumors of the lung. The tumor may appear as a single mass lesion on the x-ray film of the chest, and the diagnosis can generally be established by bronchial or transbronchial biopsy. If the tumor obstructs a bronchus, it may cause collapse of the lung. Any patient with atelectasis requires bronchoscopy to exclude cancer. An obstructing lesion may also cause persistent inflammatory changes in the distal lung, and unresolved pneumonia is another indication for bronchoscopy because of the possibility of a lung cancer.

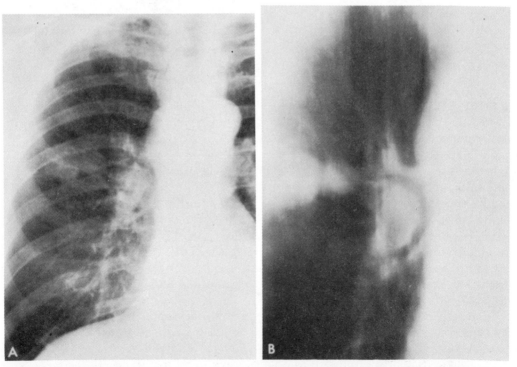

Figure 6–2 PA roentgenogram reveals a large density in the right upper lung *(A)*. On tomogram *(B)* the lesion is more clearly evident, as is the involvement of the hilum. (Reproduced with permission from Fraser, RG, and Paré, JAP: Diagnosis of Diseases of the Chest. 2nd edition. Philadelphia, W. B. Saunders Company, 1979, p. 1020.)

Figure 6–3 Cavitary lesion containing an air-fluid level that proved to be squamous cell carcinoma of the lung. (Reproduced with permission from Fraser, RG, and Paré, JAP: Diagnosis of Diseases of the Chest. 2nd edition. Philadelphia, W. B. Saunders Company, 1979, p. 1029.)

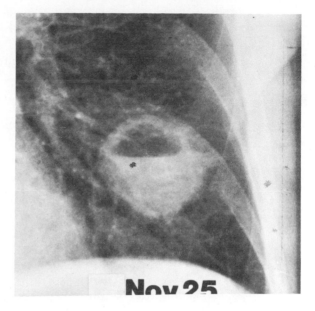

There are patients in whom bacterial pneumonia heals with cholesterol deposition in the lung, termed endogenous lipid pneumonia, which fails to change during weeks of observation. In many instances, the only way that one can be certain that the lesion is benign is to remove it. An obstructing tumor may also be associated with necrotizing pneumonia, or a tumor may grow so rapidly as to outstrip its blood supply, with resultant necrosis and abscess formation (Fig. 6–3). When a lung abscess develops in an unexpected setting, as in a patient with good oral hygiene, bronchoscopy should be done to exclude tumor as the predisposing factor.

Tumors invading the airways are very often associated with cough and frequently with hemoptysis. The onset of either of these symptoms must raise the suspicion of lung cancer, and careful radiographic study must follow. Occasionally a tumor that partially obstructs a bronchus produces characteristic slowing of a forced expiration. The normal lung empties rapidly, producing a normal FEV_1, but the obstructed lung empties slowly, causing reduction of the FEV_3. This may also be accompanied by an audible or palpable rhonchus over the affected site, particularly during a forced expiration. These signs and symptoms are useful, and they must excite the physician's suspicion. But probably the majority of patients with lung cancer have evident disease without specific symptoms.

Constitutional Symptoms

There are many ways in which carcinoma of the lung can produce constitutional symptoms. Patients with metastatic disease may present with chronic, wasting illness, or the effects of spread to one or more other organs may cause the presenting findings. Lung cancer frequently metastasizes to the brain, and it is advisable to obtain an x-ray film of the chest on any older person who develops new focal neurological findings. There have been

Table 6–1   Paraneoplastic Manifestations of Lung Cancer

Cushing's syndrome
Inappropriate secretion of ADH
Hyperparathyroidism
Gynecomastia
Pulmonary osteoarthropathy
Neuromyopathy
Carcinoid syndrome
Excessive pigmentation
Hypoglycemia

successful resections of both the primary lung cancer and the solitary cerebral metastasis, just as there have been successful resections of primary tumors elsewhere, as in the kidney, and of a solitary metastasis to the lung.

There are a great many other types of extrapulmonary symptoms, mostly associated with the release of hormonal materials from different types of lung tumors (Table 6–1). Cushing's syndrome results from tumors that produce ACTH; elaboration of antidiuretic hormone should be suspected in a patient with hyponatremia; parathormone production has caused hyperparathyroidism; and gynecomastia is probably the result of the elaboration of follicle-stimulating hormone. Finger clubbing, accompanied by the radiographic changes of pulmonary hypertrophic osteoarthropathy of the long bones, may be the presenting complaint in some patients with lung cancer and is probably due to a hormonal agent. Peripheral neuropathy, myasthenia, and even cerebellar degeneration have all occurred in patients with localized lung tumors. Bronchial adenomas are occasionally associated with the carcinoid syndrome, with characteristic episodic flushing, tremor, wheeze, diaphoresis, diarrhea, fever, and hypotension. The diagnosis is made by measuring increased amounts of serotonin or 5-hydroxy indoleacetic acid (5-HIAA) in blood or urine. Excessive pigmentation of the skin may result from elaboration of melanocyte-stimulating hormone, and production of insulin by the tumor may cause hypoglycemia. None of these findings signifies spread of the tumor or nonresectability, and the alert physician may be able to detect a small, resectable tumor in the patient who presents with such a paraneoplastic manifestation of the disease.

Direct spread of the tumor to adjacent structures may also cause the presenting complaints. Two of the most common disorders are pleural effusion and superior vena cava obstruction (SVC syndrome). Pleural effusion due to lung cancer is generally the result of invasion of the pleural surfaces by the tumor, but this is not always the case. Pleural effusion may be the result of infection that has spread from pneumonitis distal to the tumor, so that the presence of pleural effusion is not necessarily a contraindication to surgical resection. Evaluation is based on careful study of pleural fluid and tissue obtained by biopsy for malignant cells. If they cannot be found, one may consider resection.

Obstruction of the superior vena cava results in venous engorgement of the face and neck with edema, often associated with Horner's syndrome and hoarseness because of involvement of the adjacent vagus and recurrent laryngeal nerves, respectively. Such a tumor is inoperable, but the vena cava obstruction requires therapy, generally with radiation and, in some centers, with chemotherapy as well. The majority of patients with SVC syndrome have an inoperable lung cancer as the cause, but it may also result from lymphoma. Less commonly it may be the result of fibrous obstruction of the superior vena cava from previous infection, such as histoplasmosis or even tuberculosis, and it is important to obtain mediastinal tissue so as to make the diagnosis and institute appropriate therapy promptly.

Specific Syndromes

There are five kinds of tumors with such specific and interesting patterns of growth, each with important clinical implications, that they require special mention.

Lymphangitic Carcinomatosis

Some extrapulmonary neoplasms embolize to the lungs, continue to grow, and spread through the lymphatics, resulting in an extensive diffuse infiltration of the lung. Lymphangitic carcinomatosis produces progressive and severe dyspnea because of the severe restriction of lung expansion associated with the interference of gas exchange from capillary invasion. The x-ray reveals a diffuse fibronodular infiltration of the lung parenchyma, which cannot be distinguished with certainty from any form of diffuse interstitial pneumonitis, and widespread vascular occlusion may produce pulmonary hypertension with cor pulmonale. In many instances the primary tumor is not evident and the presenting complaints may be those of the pulmonary lesion.

Alveolar Cell Carcinoma

Alveolar cell carcinoma refers to tumors, similar histologically to adenocarcinoma, that characteristically grow within the alveolar spaces. They may represent a specific cell type, or they may simply be a special form of adenocarcinoma, originating either in the lung or elsewhere, since adenocarcinomas originating in other organs and metastasizing to the lung have been associated with this pattern of growth. The tumors may be localized, in which case there is a high rate of totally successful surgical resection, so that early diagnosis is important. They also may appear as disseminated lesions throughout the lung, suggestive of a bronchogenic spread, although this mechanism has not been established (Fig. 6–4). The tumors are unusual in that they may appear as areas of pneumonic infiltration, often with an air bronchogram, which are lacking in most other cases of lung cancer because of invasion of airways. In addition, the involved lung continues to be perfused because the tumors may not invade capillary walls, and a characteristic feature of bronchoalveolar carcinoma is the presence of normal or only minimally reduced perfusion on lung scan in an area of obvious disease. There are very few other conditions, one of which is alveolar proteinosis, in which lung perfusion is maintained in the face of diffuse parenchymal involvement. Most bronchogenic carcinomas are associated with such extensive involvement of blood vessels that more reduction of perfusion is evident on lung scan than would be suspected from the x-ray film of the chest.

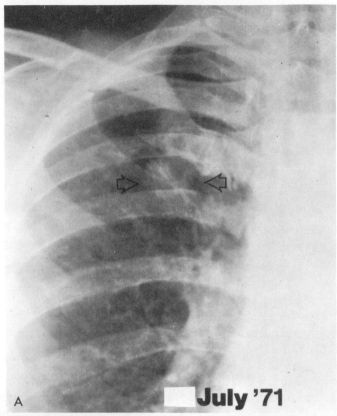

July '71

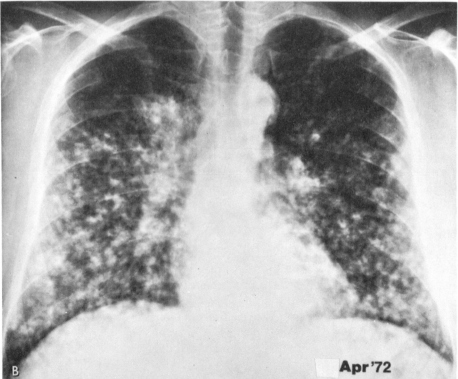

Apr '72

Figure 6–4 Small nodule in the RUL of an asymptomatic man *(A)*. Nine months later there was widespread involvement of both lungs from the alveolar cell carcinoma *(B)* Reproduced with permission from Fraser, RG, and Paré, JAP: Diagnosis of Diseases of the Chest. 2nd edition. Philadelphia, W. B. Saunders Company, 1979, p. 1062.)

Oat Cell Carcinoma

Oat cell tumors, or small cell anaplastic tumors, are biologically distinctive in that the vast majority grow so rapidly that widespread metastases are produced before symptoms become evident. If the diagnosis of oat cell carcinoma is made by transbronchial biopsy most physicians today would now employ chemotherapy, which is associated with prolonged and improved life, rather than surgery, which is almost uniformly unsuccessful. There is evidence that when oat cell tumors present as small coin lesions they can be successfully resected. But a large lesion, which can be diagnosed by transbronchial biopsy, is probably inoperable. In doubtful cases, a bone marrow examination may reveal tumor cells in about half the patients.

Papillary Formation

Bronchogenic carcinomas with a marked tendency to papillary formation seem to have the opposite, unique biological characteristic — they remain locally invasive and grow very slowly. If possible, such tumors should be resected. If this is not possible, radiotherapy, and these tumors are generally quite radiosensitive, is certainly indicated. The presence of a visible tumor on x-ray, often associated with atelectasis of the lung for a period of several years, is quite compatible with this type of lung cancer.

Pancoast Tumors

Pancoast tumors, which may be of any cell type, are tumors that arise in the superior sulcus of the lung. They also seem to have a unique biological nature in that they grow very slowly and locally (Fig. 6–5). They often present with involvement of the brachial plexus and neurological findings, having invaded the chest wall and caused rib destruction. These tumors appear to be particularly responsive to radiotherapy, and there have been a number of instances in which radiotherapy has resulted in apparent cure. Since the lesion is usually so extensive that it precludes immediate surgery, the primary treatment is radiotherapy and, if tumor size can be reduced to a manageable size, this may be followed by resection.

TREATMENT

Evaluation for Surgery

Obviously, the preferred treatment for lung cancer is total surgical excision. Unfortunately, as has been emphasized, this is so often unsuccessful that very careful evaluation of each patient is required. This must take two forms. It is necessary to make as certain as possible that the tumor is so confined that it can be removed in its entirety, and it is necessary to make sure that the patient can tolerate the resection.

The evaluation for resectability ranges from simple radiographic examination, as in a coin lesion, to far more extensive study. In most cases, tomograms and barium swallow x-rays provide the initial clues as to the extent of involvement, particularly of the mediastinum. In patients with large central lesions, pulmonary angiograms are useful in that they may

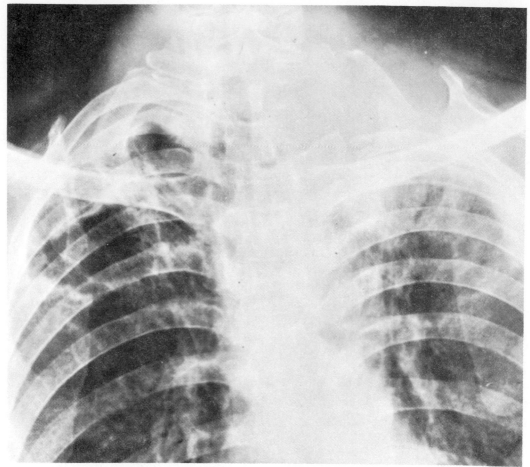

Figure 6–5 Superior sulcus tumor on the left with extensive rib destruction. (Reproduced with permission from Fraser, RG, and Paré, JAP: Diagnosis of Diseases of the Chest. 2nd edition. Philadelphia, W. B. Saunders Company, 1979, p. 1032.)

reveal invasion of the vena cava or pulmonary veins, which makes resection impossible. In doubtful cases, particularly if there is any suggestion of mediastinal involvement, tissue should be obtained from that region either by mediastinoscopy or by mediastinotomy before resection is carried out. The significance of pleural effusion with regard to resectability is noted in Chapter 7 (page 132), and careful examination for diaphragmatic paralysis, palpable supraclavicular lymph nodes, and evidence of disease in other organs is always essential.

It is now felt that asymptomatic distant metastases are so rarely detected by scanning or other procedures that the search for them is unwarranted in the absence of signs such as abnormal liver function or anemia. Thus, liver scans, brain scans, bone marrow biopsies, and bone scans are reserved for patients in whom there is reason to suspect a distant metastasis. If at all possible, the diagnosis of tumor should be made before surgery, but in small lesions this may not be possible and biopsy or even resection of the lesion may have to be performed before a definite diagnosis can be made. It is important, however, that the least possible amount of normal lung, certainly no more than a lobe, be resected until a definite tissue diagnosis has been made.

Whether or not a patient can tolerate a lung resection involves a great deal of judgment. In patients with life-limiting disease, or in patients with severe congestive heart failure or atherosclerotic heart disease, it is often felt that surgical resection would carry a prohibitive mortality. In such patients, even if the lesion is technically resectable, radiotherapy may have to be used. Lung cancer is frequently associated with chronic obstructive disease, since they both result from cigarette smoking, and it is often necessary to make a judgment as to whether or not pulmonary function is sufficient to permit resection of the lung. Again, there are no firm guidelines, but it is generally felt that if the COPD is of such severity as to produce chronic hypercapnia, lung resection cannot be tolerated.

One approach for judging the feasibility of lung resection is to assess the patient's ability to exercise; if oxygen consumption can be doubled with comfort, it is likely that significant amounts of lung may be resected without producing severe pulmonary insufficiency. Clinically evident pulmonary hypertension probably implies that so much of the pulmonary circulation has been destroyed that further reduction by surgical removal would be intolerable. Another approach is to estimate the degree of ventilatory function that the patient will have after resection. One can measure FEV_1, estimate from ventilation scans the amount of ventilated lung that will be resected, and then calculate what the FEV_1 will be after thoracotomy. An FEV_1 of 600 cc is compatible with life; and if one calculates that the postoperative FEV_1 will be 600 cc or higher, resection may be feasible.

Radiotherapy

Radiotherapy is the other major form of treatment for lung cancer, and it is certainly true that it may cause total disappearance of the tumor, particularly if confined to a single area. In disseminated disease, radiotherapy is of no more value than surgical resection, but in patients with localized, resectable disease who are not deemed candidates for surgery because of impaired pulmonary function or other medical complications radiotherapy may indeed produce cure. The value of radiotherapy in Pancoast tumors has already been noted, and it is the treatment of choice for patients with SVC syndrome. It is interesting that radiotherapy has been followed by reversal of the symptoms without recanalization of the obstructed vena cava. It is possible that radiation increases the rate of development of the collateral circulation so as to provide new pathways for venous drainage from the upper part of the body.

A number of studies have clearly shown that radiotherapy does not enhance the beneficial efforts of surgery. It should not, with the exceptions noted, be used preoperatively in order to reduce tumor bulk nor should it be used postoperatively in an effort to eradicate disease that was not resected. On the other hand, there are indications for radiotherapy in patients with nonresectable disease in whom specific symptoms develop. These include bronchial obstruction with atelectasis and distal pneumonitis and bone pain.

Palliative radiotherapy may induce symptomatic improvement of these and other conditions without improving the outlook for survival.

Other Treatment

A great effort is being made to develop regimens of chemotherapy that may be effective in the treatment of inoperable lung cancer. To date, this type of therapy has only proven effective in oat cell carcinoma, and there is clear indication now that radiotherapy can prolong survival and quality of life in this particular disease. Otherwise, chemotherapy should be considered as experimental and utilized in conjunction with an appropriately designed and supervised clinical trial.

The primary physician has a responsibility to the patient with lung cancer to provide continuing comfort and support. This includes availability to discuss the illness and its implications and to assess and hopefully treat complications as they develop. It is important not to ascribe every new illness to the tumor in a patient with inoperable disease, since such patients may well experience intercurrent treatable illness or disease, such as nosocomial infection, which is related to the treatment of the cancer. It is also important, after successful surgical therapy, to insist that the patient stop smoking, because there have been many instances in which a second or even a third primary tumor has developed. The pathological effect of cigarette smoke seems to last up to 15 years after discontinuing cigarettes. It is likely that this long a period is necessary before the patient who stops smoking can be considered no longer at risk, so that continuing surveillance is necessary for a long time after a tumor has been removed.

PREVENTION

It is clear, as already noted, that the only way to prevent lung cancer is to abolish cigarette smoking or, in some way, to render cigarettes smoke harmless. The fact that so many physicians have given up cigarettes suggests that it may be possible to reach other segments of the population if appropriate education can be provided. Unfortunately, this is not happening, and cigarette smoking continues to spread, particularly among adolescents. A wide variety of programs have been developed to discourage smoking, and most of them have been only partially successful at best. It appears that the more elaborate the program, the more successful it will be; and people who spend a great deal of time and money on giving up the smoking habit are more apt to be successful.

The other approach to the problem would be detection of lung cancer at a time when it is totally resectable. It has already been noted that efforts to do this by semiannual x-ray examination of the chest of smokers has resulted in only a slight increase in the cure rate, so that this is not a feasible approach.

Several centers are now studying radiographic detection in conjunction with cytological screening of sputum in an effort to discover disease that is curable. In fact, there are a number of patients in whom a positive cytology, even in the presence of a normal x-ray, has led to careful bronchoscopic examination with the detection of a small tumor that was successfully resected. The sputum specimen must be examined by a skilled cytologist and the bronchoscopy performed by an experienced person who can evaluate small abnormalities of the airways and obtain pathological material for study. It is not known to what extent false-positive cytology or positive cytology at a stage when the tumor cannot be detected through the broncho-scope will make this expensive approach of low cost and significant benefit. The individual who insists on smoking and yet wishes to learn about the development of lung cancer at the earliest possible stage might be well advised to enter one of these detection programs.

MEDIASTINAL TUMORS

Most mediastinal tumors are asymptomatic and are discovered on a routine chest x-ray. The location and extent of the lesion must then be determined by radiographic studies, including oblique films, tomography, and a barium swallow, which may reveal displacement or involvement of the eosphagus. Pulmonary angiography is frequently necessary to assess the relationship to the superior vena cava, aorta, and its branches and pulmonary arteries. These lesions are best considered from the standpoint of the mediastinal compartment in which they are most likely to occur.

Anterior Mediastinum

The three most common lesions of the anterior mediastinum are tumors deriving from embryonal tissue (teratomas and dermoid cysts), thymomas, and substernal goiters. Teratodermoid lesions are most common in young adults and are frequently of very large size. Thymomas may occur at any age, are often malignant, and may be associated with a number of diseases, notably myasthenia gravis but also thyrotoxicosis and Cushing's syndrome. Substernal thyroids occasionally are sufficiently functional to be diagnosed by their uptake of radioactive iodine, in which case there is no immediate indication for resection unless they produce symptoms, particularly tracheal obstruction. Otherwise, the potential for the presence of malignant disease is such that anterior mediastinal tumors should be resected once they have been localized by appropriate radiographic studies.

Middle Mediastinum

Lesions in this location most commonly involve the hilar lymph nodes either from tumor or from a more benign process. Primary carcinoma of the lung is the most common tumor involving the hilar nodes, but metastatic tumors may do the same. The hilar adenopathy associated with primary tuberculosis and sarcoidosis has been considered previously. Bronchogenic and pericardial cysts may occur in the middle mediastinum and are generally very well circumscribed and asymptomatic. Diaphragmatic hernia may appear as a mass lesion in the right cardiophrenic angle, and the diagnosis may be made by barium studies. It is rarely symptomatic and does not require surgery.

Posterior Mediastinum

Neurogenic tumors are the most common lesions in this compartment and are of sufficient malignant potential to require surgery. A variety of esophageal lesions, such as diverticuli, aneurysms of the descending aorta, paraspinal abscess (Pott's disease), and a number of other less common conditions may also occur in this location.

Additional Reading

Boucot KR, Weiss W: Is curable lung cancer detected by semi-annual screening? JAMA 224:1361–1365, 1973.
Moser KM: Solitary pulmonary nodules. JAMA 227:1167–1168, 1974.
Rodescu D: Lung Cancer. Med Clin North Am 61:1205–1218, 1977.

CHAPTER SEVEN

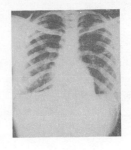

PLEURA AND CHEST WALL

Chest medicine is concerned with a great many extrapulmonary conditions that involve the chest cage and pleura. Primary care physicians should be capable of evaluating and treating acute pleurisy, they should be familiar with the characteristic features of pleural effusion, and they should be able to arrive at a tentative diagnosis by their examination of pleural fluid. They should be familiar with the effects of pleural scarring, fibrothorax, and pneumothorax, which they should be able to treat. Finally, they should be familiar with the ways in which neuromuscular and skeletal disease can restrict the lungs and how pulmonary complications can be prevented and treated.

PLEURISY

Pleuritic pain is a very common symptom, and it has several characteristic features. It is generally very abrupt in onset and so severe that it causes the patient to seek medical attention very promptly. It is usually unilateral and located in the lower and lateral areas of the chest, although it may be referred to shoulder or abdomen; it is rarely central in location. It is usually well localized and is accentuated by respiratory movements such as deep breathing or cough. It may be associated with evident splinting of the chest and with a pleural friction rub. It is most closely mimicked by musculoskeletal pain, but the latter is more often intermittent and noncontinuous and frequently bilateral and may be associated with tenderness to palpation of the overlying area of the chest. The tightness and discomfort associated with bronchitis is more central in location, although it may be accentuated by deep breathing and coughing.

Pleurisy may be the result of inflammatory changes in the pleural membranes without other evident disease, or it may be due to a variety of underlying conditions. When it occurs as an isolated event, it is most commonly due to nonbacterial infection, notably with the Coxsackie virus or other agents that cause pleurodynia. It may be associated with upper respiratory symptoms and fever, is generally self-limited, and disappears in a few days. Pulmonary emboli may cause pleuritic pain without parenchy-

127

mal disease or pleural effusion and will be discussed in Chapter 8. Herpes zoster is a common cause of unilateral segmental chest pain, which must be differentiated from acute pleurisy. It may be associated with hyperesthesia before the characteristic eruption appears.

Pleuritic pain is a common symptom or presenting complaint in a variety of other diseases. It is characteristic of pneumothorax, which is discussed later. In many instances bacterial pneumonia adjacent to the pleural surface will lead to sufficient irritation to cause pleurisy, even in the absence of an evident pleural effusion, and some patients with peripheral tumors of the lung complain of chest discomfort related to deep breathing. Pleurisy is also very common in patients with pleural effusions, to be discussed in the following section.

The evaluation of pleuritic pain always requires an x-ray film of the chest; if abnormality is present, diagnosis and treatment are directed toward it. If the roentgenogram is normal, symptomatic treatment should be given. Analgesics or even narcotics may be necessary to relieve pain. Indomethacin is said to be a particularly useful anti-inflammatory agent. In severe cases, intercostal nerve block may be necessary.

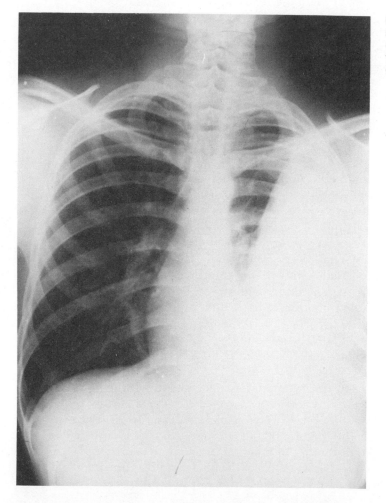

Figure 7–1 Left pleural effusion in a young man with chest discomfort. Pleural biopsy revealed caseating granuloma consistent with tuberculosis.

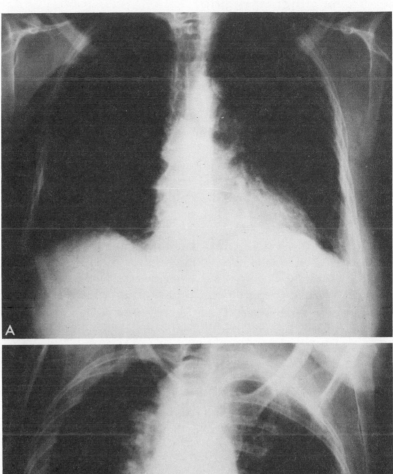

Figure 7 2 PA film of the chest with suggestion of blunting of the left costo-phrenic angle (A). Because of this finding, a decubitus film was obtained and in the right decubitus position (B) a large pleural effusion is evident tracking up into the fissure of the right lung. In the erect position (A) this fluid was collected above the diaphragm and was not visible. Sometimes such an infrapulmonic effusion is suggested by an abrupt change in density below the lung rather than the gradual transition to opacity that characterizes the normal lung.

PLEURAL EFFUSION

Although a pleural effusion is often evident because of the characteristic findings of dullness and diminished breath sounds, this is not always the case, and the diagnosis is best based on radiographic studies. To distinguish pleural thickening from free fluid, decubitus films should be obtained in order to demonstrate the layering of the fluid that occurs with effusion. In some cases of infrapulmonic effusion, the fluid may collect entirely above the diaphragm and may appear either as a pneumonic lesion at the base of the lungs or as an elevated diaphragm. An infrapulmonic effusion is suggested by the finding of an abrupt change of contrast between lung and diaphragm rather than the gradual transition that occurs as the normal lung blends into the lower portions of the diaphragm. Decubitus films can generally resolve this problem.

The first step in the evaluation of a pleural effusion is careful examination of fluid obtained by thoracentesis. This examination should include measurements of the concentration of total protein, lactic acid dehydrogenase (LDH), glucose, and amylase as well as cell count, Gram and acid-fast stains for bacteria, Wright stain for cellular morphology, cytological study, and determination of pH. Measurements of antinuclear antibodies or rheumatoid factor may be useful in patients with connective tissue disease. In patients who present as a diagnostic problem, particularly if they are not acutely ill, thoracentesis should be accompanied by a pleural biopsy for more definitive diagnostic information, since if the biopsy is not done at the time of the first tap, it may be difficult to obtain it later when there is less fluid present.

Transudates

Pleural fluid is formed and absorbed through capillaries of both the systemic (parietal pleura) and the pulmonary (visceral pleura) circulation. Although the parietal pleura seems to be dominant, pleural effusions do not occur from elevation of systemic venous pressure alone and are generally seen in patients with increased pressure in both the pulmonary and systemic veins.

Table 7-1 Some Characteristics of Pleural Effusions

Nature of the Fluid
    Grossly bloody: Trauma, malignancy, embolism
    Feculent odor: Empyema
    Milky: Chylothorax

Transudate vs. Exudate
    Specific gravity: <1.016
    Protein: Pleural/serum <0.5
    LDH: Pleural/serum <0.6

Glucose: <30 mg %: Rheumatoid disease

Elevated Amylase: Pancreatitis, esophageal rupture (markedly elevated), malignancy
pH: < 7.20. Empyema probably requires chest tube

Transudates result from either elevation of the capillary pressure or reduction of the serum oncotic pressure or both together. They are common in congestive heart failure, in hypoproteinemia associated with cirrhosis, and in renal disease and occur even after an excessive fluid overload.

Commonly, fluid has been classified as a transudate when the protein concentration is less than 3 gm per 100 ml or when the specific gravity is less than 1.016. These criteria are not strictly accurate, and it is now felt that the designation should be based upon the combination of a pleural fluid protein/serum protein of less than 0.5 and a pleural fluid LDH/serum LDH of less than 0.6. Long-standing transudation may ultimately lead to the presence of fluid that is more exudative in nature.

The cause of the transudate is generally apparent from the nature of the underlying disease, most commonly congestive heart failure. In this condition, for unknown reasons the effusion is more apt to occur on the right than the left side, and it may be of sufficient magnitude to accentuate the patient's dyspnea. For that reason, thoracentesis is often indicated to provide symptomatic relief; otherwise treatment is directed at the underlying disorder.

Parapneumonia

Pleural effusion is a common accompaniment of bacterial pneumonia, particularly pneumococcal pneumonia, which so frequently involves the periphery of the lung. It is generally wise to obtain a small sample of fluid in order to exclude serious empyema and to try to identify the infecting organism, which may not be evident from the sputum examination. Otherwise, most such effusions are of little consequence to the patient and will resolve with successful antibiotic therapy.

Pleural effusion also is a frequent accompaniment of mycoplasmic infections and, possibly, of viral pneumonia. Generally the amount of exudation is small, and it may only be possible to demonstrate the pleural effusion by obtaining x-ray films with the patient in the decubitus position.

Empyema

Frank pus in the pleural space is a much more serious problem, and empyema may appear either as the primary event or in association with evident bacterial pneumonia. Patients with rheumatoid disease appear to be particularly predisposed to the development of empyema, often recurrently. Gram stain and, ultimately, bacterial cultures are essential for institution of appropriate antibiotic therapy. In addition, it is essential to provide adequate drainage of the pleural space. If the fluid can be removed easily, thoracentesis may suffice, but often this is not possible and it is necessary to insert a chest tube in order to provide adequate drainage. The pleural fluid pH is a very useful measurement in pleural effusion associated with infection. It has been found that if the pH is less than 7.20, the fluid will not resolve without chest tube drainage.

If the infection has been present for some time, the fluid may become so loculated as to defy tube drainage, and it may be necessary to perform an open thoracotomy. Patients with empyema generally require prolonged therapy with antibiotics, often for as long as three months, although this does not require continuing hospitalization.

Tuberculosis

Tuberculous pleural effusion is still a common illness and probably ranks with carcinoma of the lung as the most common cause of pleural effusion in patients without otherwise evident disease. It is the pleural expression of the delayed hypersensitivity of tuberculosis and generally appears when the tuberculin skin test becomes positive after the initial infection. It is usually unilateral. Characteristically the fluid contains mostly lymphocytes, although in the first two weeks polymorphonuclear leukocytes may predominate. Mesothelial cells are rarely present, a feature that is sometimes of diagnostic value, and the glucose concentration is usually low. It is generally impossible to recover acid-fast organisms from the fluid, even by culture. The diagnosis is made with certainty by finding caseating granuloma, sometimes containing acid-fast organisms, by pleural biopsy. This is often not possible, however. If the tuberculin skin test is positive in patients in whom the diagnosis of tuberculosis or some other disease cannot be made, it is wise to treat as if the effusion were due to tuberculosis.

Most tuberculous effusions disappear spontaneously within a few weeks, but it has been clearly shown that they are likely to be followed by reactivation pulmonary tuberculosis at a later date. For that reason, patients with a tuberculous pleural effusion must be treated with isoniazid and ethambutol for a full year.

Cancer

Pleural effusion is frequently the presenting finding in patients with carcinoma of the lung and generally but not always indicates inoperability. The fluid is usually bloody, in contrast to a tuberculous effusion, which presents the principal diagnostic problem. Careful radiographic study, after complete drainage by thoracentesis, may reveal the primary malignancy in the lung. The effusion may be due to tumor implants within the pleura or to obstruction of lymphatics, with interruption of lymphatic drainage. Neoplastic effusions may contain malignant cells on cytological examination, or the diagnosis may be made by finding these cells on pleural biopsy. Such a finding indicates inoperability. The effusion may also result from pneumonia associated with the tumor, and if it fails to recur after thoracentesis and if malignant cells cannot be found in the fluid or pleural biopsy, the patient should be considered potentially operable.

Neoplastic disease produces a much more extensive pleural effusion than almost any other condition. The finding of total opacification of the thorax, particularly if the trachea is shifted to the side of the lesion because of collapse of the lung from the underlying tumor, is strongly suggestive of malignancy. These effusions tend to recur rapidly after they have been drained by thoracentesis, and the continuing accumulation of fluid may result in so much discomfort that therapeutic control is required. A number of agents, such as quinacrine hydrochloride (Atabrine), nitrogen mustards, and tetracycline, have been injected into the pleural space, after drainage of the fluid, in an effort to induce pleural symphysis, but this is often unsuccessful. This is more often effective if the injection is combined with rubber tube drainage, which adds mechanical irritation to the chemical effect of the drug.

Lymphomas and leukemia are frequently associated with pleural effusion, but usually late in the course after the diagnosis has been clearly established. Mesothelioma is a rare tumor arising in the pleura; it may occur as a localized growth, which is resectable, or, more commonly as a diffuse neoplasm associated with extensive pleural effusion. It is particularly common in patients who have been exposed to asbestos.

Connective Tissue Disease

Lupus erythematosus and rheumatoid arthritis are both associated with pleural effusions in a great many cases. In lupus the effusion is generally not massive; it may occur as the presenting complaint, or it may occur in association with other features of the illness. In some instances the characteristic LE cell is present in the pleural effusion, so that the diagnosis can be made. Rheumatoid arthritis is associated with pleural effusion in up to 5 per cent of patients and, as in lupus, the effusion may dominate the clinical picture and may even antedate the development of joint pain. A unique feature of rheumatoid effusion is the extremely low concentration of glucose in the fluid, often less than 20 mg%, which may be diagnostic. Rheumatoid factor may be present in the pleural effusion, and cytological elements similar to the rheumatoid nodule may be seen on pleural biopsy. Such effusions rarely require specific therapy.

Intra-Abdominal Disease

Subphrenic abscess is frequently associated with pleural effusion usually characterized by elevation or immobility of the affected diaphragm. The underlying abdominal disease should be evident. Pleural effusion is also a frequent complication of pancreatitis, and elevation of the pleural fluid amylase is characteristic.

Other Conditions

There are a great many other conditions that may present as or be associated with pleural effusion. Diffuse interstitial lung disease, notably sarcoidosis and asbestosis, is not infrequently accompanied by a pleural effusion, which poses more of a diagnostic than therapeutic problem, since it is generally asymptomatic and requires no therapy. Pleural effusion in association with ascites or ovarian carcinoma (Meigs' syndrome) may be due either to overload of pleural lymphatics by drainage of fluid from the abdomen or to an actual perforation of the diaphragm with pleural ascites. If sought for by decubitus films, a small pleural effusion can be detected in a high percentage of patients who have undergone laparotomy.

Except for *Nocardia,* which causes empyema adjacent to pulmonary suppuration, fungi do not cause pleural effusions, and the only parasitic infection associated with pleural effusion is amebiasis. Hemothorax, a bloody pleural effusion, may result from trauma or may be associated with spontaneous pneumothorax. Chylous pleural effusion results from damage to the thoracic duct, generally from trauma or tumor.

Occasionally a pleural effusion may contain a predominance of eosinophils, but they are of little diagnostic significance. They are frequently found in association with hemothorax or after a pneumothorax, but they may occur in a variety of other settings, including a viral or parapneumonic effusion. In the latter case, pleural eosinophilia is said to be a good prognostic sign, since such effusions rarely become purulent.

Rupture of the esophagus is a surgical emergency and may follow prolonged vomiting or trauma, leading to pleural effusion. It is often associated with subcutaneous and mediastinal emphysema. A very high amylase value in pleural fluid and a pH less than 6.0 are strongly suggestive of this serious illness.

FIBROTHORAX

Fibrothorax occurs when the pleural surfaces become fused by fibrous tissue, often with calcification. It is commonly the result of a previous hemothorax that has not been promptly drained, of tuberculous empyema or tuberculosis treated with pneumothorax, or of other types of empyema. It may result in such severe restriction of pulmonary function that dyspnea occurs and is generally associated with diminished respiratory movement on the affected side. The pleural thickening should be evident on the x-ray film of the chest, but severe pleural restriction may occur in the absence of a very thick pleura on the roentgenogram. Furthermore, localized pleural thickenings may produce a large lesion on the roentgenogram without much impairment of lung function.

Evaluation of fibrothorax requires measurements of lung volumes. Marked reduction of vital capacity should lead to assessment of the contribution of each lung by ventilation scans. If the restriction is due to unilateral pleural symphysis, decortication may be indicated. It is sometimes difficult to decide whether reduction of lung volumes is due to parenchymal fibrosis or pleural thickening. When there is fibrosis of the underlying lung, decortication usually fails to restore function to that lung. Fibrosis of the underlying lung can often be suspected when there was extensive lung abscess or indolent tuberculosis accompanying the empyema, but it is often difficult to ascertain the presence of parenchymal fibrosis.

Even with tomographic studies it may be impossible to distinguish between fibrotic strands and atelectasis of the trapped lung. A useful approach to this problem is to measure pleural pressure with an esophageal balloon. In severe restriction due to interstitial lung disease, lung recoil force is greatly increased and is reflected in a much more negative pleural pressure than normal. In contrast, when the lung is restricted by pleural symphysis or contraction of the chest cage, the recoil pressure is reduced rather than increased. A long duration of pleural thickening need not preclude successful surgery, and it has been shown that fibrothorax can exist for a great many years and still be corrected by decortication.

PNEUMOTHORAX

Spontaneous pneumothorax occurs when, generally in young adult males, an alveolus or emphysematous bleb ruptures into the pleural space. Air enters the pleural space until it reaches atmospheric pressure or until the collapsed lung no longer provides communication with the pleura. Normally, the negative intrapleural pressure causes both retraction of the chest cage and expansion of the lung so that as the pleural pressure rises, the chest expands at the same time as the lung collapses. For that reason, the intercostal spaces may be widened on the affected side.

Pneumothorax may be the result of trauma, either from a bronchoscope or from the outside, but it most often occurs without antecedent cause, usually at rest. It is generally characterized by sudden onset of chest pain and, then, a degree of dyspnea that is dependent upon the degree to which the lung has collapsed. There may be no symptoms if the pneumothorax is small. Physical examination may reveal hyper-resonance and decreased breath sounds on the affected side, but often these signs are absent and diagnosis is dependent upon the radiographic demonstration of air outlining the lung on the affected side. A small pneumothorax may require an expiration film to highlight the contrast between lung tissue and surrounding air. In rare instances a check-valve communication between lung and pleura permits the pneumothorax to increase during inspiration but not to empty during expiration, leading to a tension pneumothorax with collection of air under positive pressure. This causes a shift of the mediastinum to the other side, with severe dyspnea, and requires immediate relief.

If less than 25 per cent of the lung is collapsed, it may be possible simply to observe the patient to make sure that further air leakage does not occur. Ultimately, the air will be slowly absorbed, as from any closed space, owing to the fact that the air pocket is at atmospheric pressure, whereas the total pressure of gases in venous blood is lower. This is due to the fact that although arterial blood is at atmospheric pressure, having equilibrated with alveolar air, the drop of partial pressure of oxygen by uptake by the cells is much greater than the increase of Pco_2 resulting from CO_2 production. This result is reflected in the different shapes of the dissociation curves for oxygen and carbon dioxide. The rate of gas absorption can be greatly accelerated if the patient breathes pure oxygen, thus eliminating nitrogen from the blood and tissues. Under these circumstances, the pressure of gases in venous blood is the sum of the Po_2 and Pco_2, less than 100 mm Hg, and is far below atmospheric pressure, which exists in the gas pocket. This principle can also be utilized in reducing abdominal discomfort associated with intestinal obstruction. It is the reason why gas is absorbed so much more quickly from oxygen-filled than air-filled alveoli after occlusion of a bronchus, making atelectasis a common complication of oxygen breathing. Because of its toxic effects, 100 per cent oxygen is no longer used to eliminate gas pockets or stores, but 40 per cent oxygen would have some effect and should not be hazardous.

Larger pneumothoraces are generally treated by placement of a chest tube either to an underwater seal, allowing the air to be expelled by the patient's own expiratory effort and cough, or under negative pressure so that the lung can be expanded by aspiration of the air. After expansion has occurred, the tube can be clamped, generally within 1 to 2 days, and if the lung remains expanded, the tube can be withdrawn. A totally collapsed lung should not be expanded completely at once, since this may lead to the formation of pulmonary edema, probably as the result of sudden restoration of the circulation to a previously collapsed capillary bed. Pneumothorax may be associated with pleural bleeding (hemothorax), in which case it is important to insert a chest tube to evacuate the blood and prevent the development of pleural fibrosis. If a thoracic surgeon is not present and appropriate facilities are not available, it is possible for the physician to insert a small plastic catheter in an anterior upper interspace with the patient semirecumbent so as to provide lung expansion. It is better to do this through a catheter than through a needle in order to prevent injury to the lung as it expands and reaches the pleural surface. The same technique may be used for the aspiration of a pleural effusion.

Most pneumothoraces are not associated with pre-existing lung disease, but they can occur in individuals with diffuse lung diseases, notably histiocytosis X, that are associated with subpleural blebs or bullae. If, however, one performs a thoracotomy on a patient with pneumothorax, it is generally possible to identify a small subpleural bleb indicative of the predisposing lesion. Pulmonary function studies on patients who have had pneumothorax have revealed no abnormality showing that it is not a result of generalized emphysema but, rather, of a very localized disease.

In most instances there is no disability following re-expansion of the lung, but in a small percentage of patients the pneumothorax may recur. If this happens more than once, it is probably wise to perform a thoracotomy and induce symphysis between parietal and visceral pleura by mechanical abrasion. If blebs or bullae are present, they may be resected. Bilateral pneumothorax is an indication for pleurodesis on at least one side to avoid possibly fatal recurrence.

NEUROMUSCULAR DISEASE

Extensive paralysis of the respiratory muscles can lead to significant impairment of respiratory function. Guillain-Barré syndrome, botulism, myasthenia gravis, and poliomyelitis can all cause rapidly progressive respiratory weakness with ventilatory failure, as discussed in Chapter 9. Chronic neuromuscular disease associated with muscular dystrophy or spinal cord disease, as in amyotrophic lateral sclerosis, can lead to substantial weakness of respiratory muscles with, in some cases, hypoventilation. Since lung mechanics are relatively normal in these conditions, artificial ventilation is easily provided, and there are some patients who can be managed quite well with a cuirass or a tank respirator. In some instances, just sleeping in the respirator provides sufficient ventilatory support to maintain arterial blood gases at normal levels. Patients with these disorders are unable to take deep breaths, so that they are particularly prone to atelectasis and respiratory infection. It is probably wise for them to use IPPB regularly, at least four times a day, preferably every hour in order to inflate the lung periodically, promote expansion of airspaces, and aid in the expectoration of sputum. Respiratory infections must be promptly detected and treated with appropriate antibiotics.

Other neurological lesions may be associated with pulmonary complications. A cerebral vascular accident may involve the respiratory muscles, but this is generally of little significance. The obtunded patient requires special attention to nasal tracheal suctioning in the event of a respiratory infection such as pneumonia. Patients with Parkinson's disease may have difficulty with coughing and seem to be quite prone to the development of pneumonia, though it usually responds well to antibiotics and vigorous physical therapy.

Diaphragmatic Paralysis

Occasionally one diaphragm may become paralyzed, with about 20 per cent reduction of ventilatory function. This is of no clinical consequence and is often asymptomatic. It is usually of unknown etiology, though it may reflect peripheral neuritis in association with infection. Unilateral elevation of the diaphragm must always raise the suspicion of phrenic nerve involvement by a bronchogenic tumor. Congenital elevation of the diaphragm, eventration, is uncommon and of no consequence except that it may be confused with phrenic paralysis.

Bilateral diaphragmatic paralysis, a rare disorder, does cause impairment of ventilatory function such that the patient may not be able to lie down and may only be able to breathe adequately in an erect position when the diaphragm is lowered by gravity, permitting better ventilation of the lungs with the intercostal muscles. Diaphragmatic paralysis may be suspected when paradoxical inward movement of the abdomen is observed on inspiration, on one side when the lesion is unilateral. The diagnosis is usually considered when the chest x-ray reveals elevation of the diaphragm, but it can only be diagnosed with certainty by fluoroscopic or cinefluorographic demonstration of paradoxical motion.

It is possible that patients with respiratory muscle weakness might improve with concentrated efforts at endurance training of the respiratory muscles, but such an approach needs more extensive development and study.

SKELETAL ABNORMALITIES

Scoliosis

Scoliosis is lateral curvature of the spine, which may occur in the thoracic region. It usually develops in childhood, and it may be associated with a variety of congenital abnormalities of the spine or it may be the result of a paralytic disease such as poliomyelitis. Mild deformities are not associated with substantial impairment of lung function, although there may be some reduction of lung volumes. Surgical correction, by insertion of Harrington rods, is generally done for cosmetic reasons. There is evidence that such a procedure is followed by increased lung volumes, paralleling the increased height resulting from growth, but the disease should be looked upon as a cosmetic rather than physiological disturbance.

Severe scoliosis with rotation of the spine and prominence of the posterior angles of the rib leading to the hunchback appearance, commonly called kyphoscoliosis, is associated with substantial impairment of lung function. The greater the angulation of the spine, the greater the compression of the underlying lung, with reduction of lung volumes. The surprising fact is that severe deformity from kyphoscoliosis, with an x-ray appearance of very little functioning lung, may be associated with relatively little disability and even a very long life.

Marked reduction of lung volumes is associated with so much increase in the work of breathing that CO_2 retention develops. In addition, the compressed lung is relatively more perfused than ventilated, leading to hypoxemia. These disturbances of arterial blood gases may be associated with pulmonary hypertension, cor pulmonale, and right-sided congestive heart failure. In addition, patients with kyphoscoliosis are very prone to the development of respiratory infection, which can lead to worsening of arterial blood gases and respiratory failure.

Treatment is directed at maintaining optimal lung inflation, and it has been shown that administration of IPPB three or four times a day is of distinct value in this condition by opening airways and reversing the atelectasis which otherwise occurs. Hypoxic patients may benefit from chronic oxygen therapy in order to minimize polycythemia and congestive heart failure, and respiratory infections must be vigorously treated with antibiotics as well as physical measures designed to induce cough and deep breathing.

Pectus Excavatum

Like simple scoliosis, a funnel-chest deformity is more of a cosmetic than physiological problem. Because of the inward displacement of the chest, the x-ray film may suggest cardiac enlargement. A systolic ejection murmur may be heard but it is of no consequence. There is usually minimal, if any, reduction of pulmonary function, and surgical correction is indicated for cosmetic reasons only.

OBESITY

Since the original description by Charles Dickens, the Pickwickian syndrome has excited considerable interest and study. Some very obese patients suffer from chronic hypercapnia and from excessive somnolence. At one time, it was felt that the somnolence was the result of hypercapnia, but it is now known that this is not the case in most instances. Hypercapnia has traditionally been ascribed to the excess work of breathing, and it is likely that a major component of this is the obese abdomen, which produces upward displacement and stretch of the diaphragm. In addition, the weight of the abdominal and thoracic contents requires extra work from the muscles of respiration, which may not be sustained. It is for this reason that when ventilatory failure develops, the obese patient should be treated in the upright position in a chair to minimize the work of breathing.

It is puzzling that all very obese patients do not show hypoventilation and that some patients who are not terribly obese do. It has been suggested that the hypoventilation syndrome in obesity is the result of at least two factors — the extra work of breathing and ineffective diaphragmatic function coupled with reduced central drive to respiration from the respiratory center. It is known that respiratory sensitivity is extremely variable, some individuals reacting vigorously with hyperventilation to small concentrations of inhaled carbon dioxide and others reacting very much less. It may be that the obese patients who develop hypoventilation are those who were born with a relatively unresponsive respiratory center. It is also possible that, in some individuals, hypothalamic damage, as from a viral infection in infancy, may lead to the excessive hyperphagia that produces obesity and to suppression of ventilation. Obese patients who smoke and develop obstructive pulmonary disease are more at risk of developing hypoventilation than are others.

In addition to the increased work of breathing, the abdominal obesity, with upper displacement of the diaphragm, causes compression of the inferior portions of the lung, which remain relatively perfused and contribute hypoxic blood to the arterial system. This is the cause of the hypoxemia in the condition that contributes to the development of cor pulmonale and congestive heart failure. It is also minimized by having the patient sit in a chair rather than lie in a bed.

The other main feature of the Pickwickian syndrome is hypersomnolence. This is not closely correlated with the degree of hypercapnia, and in recent years it has been shown that patients with obesity who fall asleep are actually suffering from sleep deprivation. It turns out that these individuals have dysfunction of the upper airways. During inspiration, there is either imperfect contraction of the genioglossus, which keeps the tongue from falling back and obstructing the airway, or abnormal contraction of other glossopharyngeal muscles with narrowing of the pharynx. As a result, these patients develop airway occlusion when they sleep, and they snore loudly and wake suddenly with a startle after a period of apnea. The continuous sleep deprivation is the cause of the daytime somnolence. It is not known why this syndrome is particularly common among obese people. It may have to do with the increase of fatty tissue in the neck, and it may be reversed by weight loss.

The *sleep apnea syndrome* is not confined to obese subjects, but it is much more common in people who are at least overweight and have short necks. It is not necessarily associated with hypercapnia, since ventilation is maintained during the wakeful state. Family members may call attention to the very loud snoring, which is always present, and to the restless sleep that the patient experiences. These patients commonly suffer from polycythemia because of the frequent periods of severe hypoxemia occurring during sleep and from hypertension, both of which are reversed by effective treatment of the sleep apnea. Other than weight reduction, tracheostomy is the only treatment currently available for this condition. A permanent tracheostomy may be opened during the night, to allow comfortable sleep, but closed during the day to permit talking and normal activities. It is followed by reversal of all the symptoms, including polycythemia and hypertension.

Severe obesity may be associated with acute ventilatory failure and will be discussed further in Chapter 9. Chronic hypercapnia is best reversed by weight reduction, but obesity is a malignant disease and very difficult to treat. Some have resorted to aggressive surgical approaches, such as wiring of the jaw and by-pass of the intestines, and these procedures may be warranted in the patient with severe physiological impairment. Other measures that may be useful include sleeping in the erect position, oxygen therapy at night in patients with polycythemia or in those who have been shown to develop nocturnal hypoxemia, and treatment of congestive failure with diuretics. It has also been shown that the administration of progesterone, which is known to stimulate ventilation during the progestational phase of the normal menstrual cycle, produces some increased ventilation in these patients, as it does in some patients with chronic hypercapnia due to obstructive pulmonary disease. This drug is more likely to be effective in obesity because the mechanical impairment of ventilation is less than it is in COPD.

Additional Reading

Guenter CA: Abnormalities of the chest walls. *In* Guenter CA, Welch MH (eds): Pulmonary Medicine. Philadelphia, J. B. Lippincott, 1977.

Light, RW: Pleural effusions. Med Clin North Am 61:1339–1352, 1977.

Pierce AK: Pleural disease. *In* Guenter CA, Welch MA (eds): Pulmonary Medicine. Philadelphia, J. B. Lippincott, 1977.

Sutton FD, Zwillich CW, Creagh CE, et al: Progesterone for outpatient treatment of Pickwickian syndrome. Ann Intern Med 83:476–479, 1975.

Walsh RE, Michaelson ED, Harkleroad LE, et al: Upper airway obstruction in obese patients with sleep disturbances and somnolence. Ann Intern Med 76:185–192, 1972.

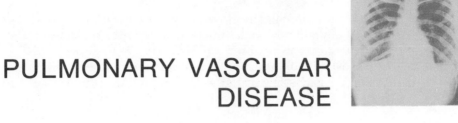

CHAPTER EIGHT

PULMONARY VASCULAR DISEASE

The pulmonary circulation is notably different from the systemic circulation in that it is designed to expose the entire cardiac output to alveolar gas over the widest possible surface area. There is little need to vary the blood flow to different parts of the lung so that, in contrast to the muscular systemic vessels, which make it possible to divert the circulation to the organs that most need it, the pulmonary vessels are relatively thin and offer low resistance to flow. The vascular bed is so large that it must be extensively obstructed before pulmonary hypertension develops. When this occurs, the underlying disease dominates the clinical picture, and the physician should understand pulmonary hypertension mainly in order to recognize the diseases that produce it and to provide appropriate treatment for them. Although the diagnosis and treatment of pulmonary embolism is an important responsibility of the primary care physician, many patients with chronic pulmonary hypertension will require specialized study.

All physicians are very familiar with pulmonary edema consequent to left ventricular failure, but many are less familiar with the growing number of cases of noncardiac pulmonary edema resulting from shock, trauma, drugs, and a host of other causes outlined in this chapter. Primary care physicians must be aware of these disorders so that they can make the diagnosis early and refer the patient to specialized facilities for appropriate care, and they must be aware of precipitating causes that may be avoided.

PULMONARY EMBOLISM

Pathogenesis

Pulmonary embolism is probably very common. It is likely that clots form in pelvic and deep leg veins rather often, even in normal people, migrate to the lungs, and are lysed by a potent fibrinolytic system present in the pulmonary circulation. Intravascular coagulation is promoted by changes in the clotting properties of the blood, by stasis, and by endothelial injury. A hypercoagulable state occurs after trauma, after surgery, and in some patients with malignant disease. Stasis is common in congestive heart failure and after

141

prolonged immobilization, such as in bed rest or sitting in a bus or car for several hours. Endothelial injury may occur in sepsis or trauma and may be the site of clot formation.

Most pulmonary embolisms originate from thrombi in the deep veins of the leg or pelvis, particularly the former. After the thrombi form they may become detached and may float in various sizes to the lung. If the patient survives, small clots are apt to be lysed by fibrinolytic enzymes in the blood. Larger clots tend to fragment and disperse peripherally where they may organize or be lysed. Recurrent pulmonary embolization leads to gradually progressive occlusion of the small blood vessels of the lung and to pulmonary hypertension.

Pathophysiology

The physiological changes that occur in the heart and the lungs, in both man and experimental animals, after pulmonary embolization have been studied in great detail. One of the first signs is the development of rapid shallow breathing, which is ascribed to stimulation of intravascular receptors, in both small and large vessels, leading to hyperventilation. This results in reduction of the arterial Pco_2. Hypocapnia is one of the most regular features of pulmonary embolism.

The remaining changes follow from occlusion of the pulmonary circulation. This is largely mechanical, but there is evidence that vasoactive amines released from blood clots may cause some pulmonary vasoconstriction. Reflex vasoconstriction, once a popular theory, no longer appears to be an important feature of this condition. Occlusion of the pulmonary circulation leads to an immediate increase in pulmonary artery pressure, but this tends to decline slowly over the next several hours as other vessels in the lung open to accommodate blood flow.

It has been shown that even after massive embolism with glass beads, which do not dissolve, severe pulmonary hypertension disappears in a few days as the pulmonary circulation expands. There is evidence that the occlusion of blood vessels is associated with some constriction of airways, particularly alveolar ducts, with reduction of ventilation. The net result of these regional changes of circulation and ventilation is the development of some units that are grossly underperfused with respect to ventilation and other units in which the perfusion exceeds ventilation. The existence of these units of differing $\dot{V}/\dot{Q}$ ratio causes fall of arterial oxygen tension. Because of hyperventilation, the arterial oxygen tension may not be terribly low, but measurements of the alveolar arterial (A-a) oxygen gradient will always reveal abnormality.

The natural course of clinical and experimental emboli is resolution, with ultimate restoration of a normal circulation unless further embolization occurs. It is for this reason that maintenance of the circulation even after extensive pulmonary embolization may be followed by full improvement and total recovery.

In the normal lung, embolic occlusion of a blood vessel does not produce pulmonary infarction, presumably because the tissue can be adequately nourished by the bronchial collateral circulation. Pulmonary infarction does occur if there is elevation of the pulmonary venous pressure, causing additional stasis. The reasons for this are not clear, but the high venous pressure may cause hemorrhage into the alveoli, causing the radiographic density characteristic of infarction. It should be noted that infarction is of little practical consequence. It usually resolves spontaneously or, rarely, heals with formation of a thin-walled cavity. There is no reliable clinical indication of pulmonary infarction other than the x-ray film of the chest. Hemoptysis is more common in patients with such a lesion than in those without, as is pleuritic chest pain, but neither of these symptoms is pathognomonic or invariably present.

Aside from an increase of the alveolar arterial oxygen tension gradient, there is little measurable disturbance of lung function. Lung volumes are generally preserved, the diffusing capacity is usually normal or only slightly reduced because there is so much extra alveolar capillary surface available for diffusion, and lung mechanics may be normal. Sensitive tests often reveal narrowing of small airways, and there have been reports that pulmonary embolism may be associated with wheezing because of bronchoconstriction. Bronchoconstriction is known to occur in the experimental animal after lobar embolization, probably a homeostatic adjustment designed to reduce ventilation to poorly perfused lungs in order to keep $\dot{V}/\dot{Q}$ ratios as near normal as possible. But this is not a prominent feature of pulmonary embolism in humans, and audible wheeze is extremely uncommon, if it occurs at all, in patients who are otherwise free of chronic lung disease.

Ultimately sustained pulmonary hypertension may lead to pulmonary edema, perhaps because a very few capillaries are now overperfused at a high pressure, perhaps because of increased permeability of the lung capillaries secondary to the widespread vascular occlusion.

Clinical Features

Despite a wealth of knowledge about and understanding of pulmonary function and the development of a great many new tests for studies of pulmonary and venous circulation, pulmonary embolism remains one of the most difficult clinical problems faced by the physician. It may occur without any symptoms at all, it may be associated with a short-lasting atrial arrhythmia, and it may cause sufficient pulmonary hypertension to lead to the abrupt onset of hyperventilation and a sense of dyspnea. A subpleural embolus may lead to sufficient pleural irritation to cause pleuritic pain, and pulmonary infarction may be associated with hemoptysis. Thus, there is a broad range of symptoms, ranging from transient breathlessness with or without pleuritic chest pain to frank hemoptysis, depending in part upon the size of the embolus and the extent of infarction.

It is extremely important to search for risk factors in patients presenting with any of these symptoms, and one must ask about a period of immobilization in the past and search for evidence of deep vein thrombosis, such as increased calf circumference or pain on pressure. The cuff test may be useful in revealing pain in one calf at a lower inflation pressure of a sphygmomanometer cuff than the other.

Most patients with documented pulmonary embolism do reveal some abnormality on the x-ray film of the chest, but this is nonspecific. Elevation of the diaphragm, pleural effusion, linear atelectasis resulting from bronchial occlusion, and areas of consolidation may all be seen, but the x-ray film may be entirely normal. In extensive embolization sufficient pulmonary hypertension is present to produce right-axis deviation on the electrocardiogram; the second pulmonic sound is accentuated, and there may be a gallop rhythm.

Just as the signs and symptoms are nonspecific and inconstant, so too are most of the laboratory tests. Only a minority of patients reveal elevation of the serum LDH, and although the diagnosis is extremely unlikely in a patient with a normal A-a gradient, the characteristic hypocapnia and reduction of arterial Po_2 are totally nonspecific. Finding a normal A-a gradient, however, may be useful in distinguishing anxiety hyperventilation from pulmonary embolism.

The perfusion lung scan has become increasingly important in the assessment of patients suspected of having this condition. It is probably true that a normal scan essentially rules out major pulmonary embolism. However, the perfusion defect characteristic of embolism also occurs in almost any other kind of lung disease, including asthma, obstructive lung disease, and most types of infiltrative pneumonic disease. Simultaneous performance of a ventilation scan is useful in that many chronic pulmonary diseases are associated with simultaneous reduction of ventilation and perfusion, and preservation of ventilation in the area of perfusion defect is much more suggestive of pulmonary embolism than the simple demonstration of absent perfusion.

In a patient with characteristic symptoms, with a normal x-ray film of the chest, a clinical diagnosis may be made by finding the characteristic abnormalities on ventilation/perfusion scan. In most patients, however, a firm diagnosis can only be made by angiography with the actual demonstration of filling defects in the pulmonary vessels. It is likely that small emboli that are not evident on the angiogram can produce hemodynamic disturbances, but it is generally felt that a positive diagnosis can only be made with characteristic angiographic findings. Some believe that anticoagulation should be reserved only for such patients. In one series, patients with the characteristic clinical features of pulmonary embolism and abnormalities on ventilation/perfusion scan but normal angiograms were not treated with anticoagulants. They suffered no further disease; if they did have emboli, they apparently did not require treatment.

Recently, attention has been directed towards the detection of deep vein thrombosis in the legs in evaluating patients for pulmonary emboli. Impedance plethysmography and Doppler ultrasound are noninvasive techniques that are useful in this regard. False-negatives and false-positives can occur with either of these tests, but if both are positive, it is extremely likely that deep vein thrombosis is present. Radio-iodine-tagged fibrinogen was found to be a sensitive marker of increased thrombosis in legs in studies carried out in Europe. Angiography of leg veins is also useful in demonstrating occlusion of deep veins, but the procedure itself causes a high incidence of local thrombophlebitis at the injection site. Other techniques, such as blood assays for fibrinopeptides, may ultimately prove extremely useful in defining patients with excessive coagulation who are at risk of developing pulmonary embolism.

A particular problem is posed by massive pulmonary embolism with occlusion of over 50 per cent of the pulmonary circulation. Such patients present characteristically with systemic hypotension and marked elevation of the venous pressure, a rather unique clinical combination that should lead to immediate suspicion of the diagnosis. Older patients with underlying disease may develop a less dramatic picture from major obstruction of the pulmonary circulation, and patients at risk must always be suspected of this complication when they develop increasing signs of right-sided heart failure or new atrial arrhythmias. The diagnosis of massive pulmonary embolization can be confirmed by finding major pulmonary hypertension with a normal pulmonary capillary wedge pressure, although absolute diagnosis requires angiography.

Treatment

The appropriate treatment of pulmonary embolism is anticoagulation. There is no doubt that patients with a significant degree of embolization are at great risk of dying from recurrent episodes and that this risk is markedly reduced by appropriate anticoagulation. Heparin should be started immediately, preferably at a dose sufficient to maintain the partial thromboplastin time between 1.5 and 2.5 times the control. If the drug is given continuously by the intravenous route, there may be fewer bleeding complications than when it is given intermittently. Oral anticoagulants are begun at the same time to maintain the prothrombin time between 2 and 2.5 times the control. At this point the heparin therapy may be discontinued. How long anticoagulation should be continued is still uncertain, but there is now evidence that if patients are maintained on anticoagulants for four months, and perhaps the interval could be shorter, they are not at risk of suffering recurrent embolization. Anticoagulants should be continued if risk factors predisposing to deep vein thrombosis continue to be present.

The presence of hypoxemia should be treated with oxygen, and analgesia may be necessary because of marked pain, dyspnea, or apprehension. During the acute phase of pulmonary embolism the patient should be monitored and cardiac arrhythmias promptly treated.

Massive pulmonary embolism with systemic hypotension requires maintenance of blood pressure with intravenous pressors such as isoproterenol, and a few centers with appropriate experience and facilities may consider a patient with persistent shock and venous hypertension for emergency embolectomy. This procedure carries a very high mortality and is not widely employed, particularly since the natural history of pulmonary embolism is in the direction of spontaneous improvement with eventual recovery. There have been reports of patients with total circulatory collapse being maintained with manual chest compression for several hours with ultimate recovery. Such maneuvers have been shown in experimental animals actually to fragment the blood clots in the right ventricle and major pulmonary arteries so that they become dispersed, with restoration of the pulmonary circulation.

Treatment with urokinase is associated with slight improvement in the rate of clearing of pulmary emboli, but there is no significant reduction of mortality and a fairly high incidence of hemorrhagic complications, so that this form of therapy has not been widely adopted.

In some patients with gastrointestinal or other types of bleeding in whom anticoagulants are contraindicated, it may be necessary to consider other approaches. One of these is the insertion of an umbrella filter into the inferior vena cava to prevent further embolization to the lungs. An alternative approach is ligation or plication of the vena cava directly. Such an approach, which may also be considered in patients with recurrent embolization while on adequate anticoagulants, is reasonable and is probably associated with less recurrent disease than would otherwise occur.

Pulmonary emboli may also occur from other sources. Thrombophlebitis with septic embolization is a common complication in intravenous drug users and is characteristically associated with multiple lesions of the lung, with necrotizing pneumonia that quickly leads to cavity formation. In this situation, treatment is with antibiotics, and anticoagulants are not felt to be of value. Such patients frequently have bacterial endocarditis and should be treated accordingly.

Tumors may also embolize to the lung, producing widespread occlusion of the pulmonary capillaries and a roentgenogram that either looks relatively normal or suggests diffuse interstitial disease. Multiple tumor emboli cause pulmonary hypertension with tachypnea and severe dyspnea. The distinction between tumor emboli and pulmonary emboli with blood clots can be made by finding a very low diffusing capacity for carbon monoxide, which is associated with tumor emboli. In this situation the tumor actually grows through the capillaries, interfering with gas exchange; whereas the pulmonary capillary bed, and the diffusing capacity, are normal after proximal obstruction by blood clots.

Fat or bone marrow embolization may follow trauma, and embolization has also occurred with amniotic fluid, air, parasites, and foreign bodies that have worked their way into the circulation from distal sites.

The general principle of treatment of pulmonary embolism is support until spontaneous resolution occurs and prevention of recurrence, which is the main indication for anticoagulation.

Prophylaxis

Prophylaxis is also important for patients who have not yet had pulmonary emboli. Deep vein thrombosis is treated with anticoagulants, and patients at risk of developing this problem can be treated with low doses of heparin — 5,000 units subcutaneously two to three times a day. Such treatment has been shown to prevent pulmonary embolism after surgery and is probably indicated for other patients at risk, such as patients with chronic obstructive pulmonary disease and ventilatory failure, individuals at bed rest after myocardial infarction or because of congestive failure, and patients over 40 undergoing elective surgery. This is not effective for established thrombotic disease and is not a substitute for adequate anticoagulation, but it is a safe, effective, prophylactic measure. Other risk factors such as immobility can be treated by appropriate movement, and leg exercises are useful in patients forced to sit for long periods of time.

Table 8–1   Pulmonary Hypertension

Chronic Obstructive Pulmonary Disease
Diffuse Lung Disease
Cardiac Disease
    Congenital
    Acquired
Pulmonary Vascular Disease
    Embolism
    Primary Pulmonary Hypertension
    Veno-Occlusive Disease

PULMONARY HYPERTENSION

An important characteristic of the pulmonary circulation is its very large reserve. At rest, only a few of the pulmonary vessels are perfused with blood, and many more are opened by increased blood flow. During exercise, the increased cardiac output can be accommodated with very little increase of the pulmonary artery pressure. In addition, progressive encroachment upon the pulmonary circulation by disease is associated with significant rise of pulmonary artery pressure only when the vascular bed is reduced to a very small fraction of that originally present. For example, embolic occlusion of pulmonary vessels only causes severe pulmonary hypertension when about 75 per cent of the circulation is occluded, and 75 per cent of the lung can be resected without overwhelming increase of the pulmonary artery pressure. Thus, advanced disease must be present before pulmonary hypertension develops, but in most cases the underlying problem presents clinical features requiring treatment long before that happens.

Pulmonary hypertension may be reflected in abnormal physical findings. The pulmonic second sound is accentuated, a palpable right ventricular heave may be present, and systemic congestion is reflected in distension of neck veins and, ultimately, edema. The roentgenogram may reveal right ventricular enlargement, and the central pulmonary arteries are prominent. Precise evaluation requires right-heart catheterization, and this, coupled with measurement of the wedge pressure, makes it possible to define the site of the obstruction, whether at or distal to the small vessels in the lung.

The major result of pulmonary hypertension is an increased load on the right ventricle, leading to increased end diastolic pressure reflected in elevation of the right atrial pressure, systemic venous congestion, and, ultimately, edema. Treatment with digitalis is of very little value, but diuretics are extremely useful in controlling edema. The main emphasis of treatment should be on the underlying disease.

The principal causes of pulmonary hypertension are listed in Table 8–1, and since they evolve in different and interesting ways, they will be considered separately.

Chronic Obstructive Pulmonary Disease

COPD is the most common cause of pulmonary hypertension. Although there is some reduction of the vascular bed, particularly in patients with extensive emphysema, the principal cause of the increased pulmonary artery pressure is the combination of hypoxemia and hypercapnia. Both increase of P_{CO_2} and reduction of arterial P_{O_2} cause increased pulmonary vascular resistance, presumably because of vasoconstriction in the small pulmonary arteries, and the effect is even greater when the two stimuli are combined. In addition, there is evidence that continuing hypoxia leads to other changes in the pulmonary arteries, including smooth muscle thickening, which leads to further increase of the pulmonary artery pressure. People living at high altitude show slight increase of pulmonary artery pressure on acute exposure, and sustained residence may be associated with vascular changes leading to more severe pulmonary hypertension. The same is true of chronic lung disease with hypoxia.

The pulmonary hypertension associated with COPD is best treated by restoring arterial blood gas composition to as near normal as possible. In patients with severe disease, prolonged oxygen therapy may be associated with considerable improvement. The administration of oxygen leads to some reduction of pulmonary pressure immediately, and continuing treatment is followed by even more pronounced improvement. If the measures aimed at treating the COPD are insufficient to correct hypoxemia, prolonged oxygen therapy should be considered. Patients with pulmonary hypertension may profit from just breathing oxygen at night in order to prevent the episodic hypoxemia that is so common. It is probably wise to institute oxygen therapy in a hospital in order to make certain that it is not associated with respiratory depression and hypercapnia.

Diffuse Lung Disease

Unlike COPD, diffuse interstitial disease of the lung produces pulmonary hypertension by direct encroachment on the pulmonary vessels by the inflammatory process and scarring. Thus, the degree of pulmonary hypertension is not related to arterial blood gas abnormality, as it is in COPD, and it is less reversible with therapy. On the other hand, it only occurs in patients with widespread disease. This is best reflected in the measurement of the diffusing capacity, which correlates inversely with the pulmonary artery pressure. The diffusing capacity is a measure of the overall capacity of the pulmonary vascular bed to exchange gases; when this bed is obliterated, there is proportional reduction of the diffusing capacity.

It has been shown, in sarcoidosis, that a reduction of the diffusing capacity to half normal is always accompanied by some increase in pulmonary artery pressure and that further reduction is associated with severe elevation of the pulmonary artery pressure. In most patients there is also reduction of lung volume, but there are exceptions, and there have been reports of patients with diffuse interstitial lung disease with pulmonary hypertension in whom the vital capacity was nearly normal. In diffuse lung disease, pulmonary hypertension indicates relatively advanced disease and a relatively poor prognosis, but treatment is directed at the underlying disease, perhaps with corticosteroids, with the use of diuretics to minimize systemic congestion.

Cardiac Disease

Congenital heart disease, in which the pulmonary circulation is overper-fused by large left-to-right shunts, is associated with anatomic changes of the pulmonary vessels, leading to increased pulmonary vascular resistance and pulmonary hypertension. The diagnosis is usually evident from the physical and radiographic examination, coupled with cardiac catheterization and angiocardiography. Acquired heart disease, notably mitral stenosis, is also associated with changes of the pulmonary vessels, probably because of the continuing stimulus of the increased capillary pressure resulting from the elevation of pressure in the pulmonary veins. Thus, the pulmonary artery pressure is elevated not only because of elevation of left atrial pressure but, in addition, because the pulmonary vascular resistance is increased by damage to the pulmonary vessels.

Pulmonary Vascular Disease

Pulmonary hypertension from primary disease of the pulmonary circulation is most commonly the result of pulmonary embolism. Massive embolization involving more than half of the pulmonary circulation produces pulmonary hypertension acutely, and recurrent embolization may ultimately lead to pulmonary hypertension when widespread occlusion of the circulation develops. The important treatment is prevention, and the diagnosis and treatment with anticoagulants were discussed previously.

Primary Pulmonary Hypertension

Primary pulmonary hypertension is a rare disease in which the primary pathology appears to be within the small pulmonary arteries, leading to muscular hypertrophy and narrowing and occlusion of the vessels. This condition has been associated with a variety of systemic diseases, including collagen vascular disease, chronic active hepatitis, and the ingestion of certain drugs, notably some anorexigens. In most of the cases the etiology remains unknown. There is a counterpart to this in the experimental production of pulmonary hypertension in animals who ingest certain al-kaloids from the weed Crotalaria. Primary pulmonary hypertension is more common among young women than men, and it is often associated with increase of serum globulins and with Raynaud's phenomenon. A variety of vasodilators have been used for treatment, and there have been recent reports that hydralazine causes reduction of pulmonary artery pressure. But the effects of these drugs are unpredictable, and they should not be used without careful hemodynamic study to make certain that they are exerting a favorable effect. There is no evidence that anticoagulants are of value, although it is extremely difficult to be certain that the condition is not the result of recurrent pulmonary embolization. In doubtful cases chronic anticoagulation may be needed. Recently, there has been a report that nocturnal oxygen therapy is associated with reduction of pulmonary hyper-tension, presumably by preventing hypoxemia or by inducing vasodilation during sleep, and this innocuous form of treatment should be evaluated more extensively.

Primary Veno-Occlusive Disease

Just as pulmonary vascular changes may result from the pulmonary congestion of left heart failure or mitral stenosis, so may occlusion of the pulmonary veins cause elevation of the pulmonary artery pressure out of proportion to the increased venous pressure. Primary veno-occlusive disease is a very rare disorder and can only be diagnosed with certainty by lung biopsy but might be suggested in a patient with unexplained pulmonary hypertension associated with Kerley B lines on the x-ray film of the chest. In addition, fibrosing mediastinitis, which may be the result of histoplasmosis or even tuberculosis, can cause pulmonary venous obstruction, as can tumors or thrombi in the left atrium.

PULMONARY ARTERIOVENOUS FISTULA

Pulmonary arteriovenous (AV) fistula is a rare defect of the pulmonary circulation in which there is a direct communication between a pulmonary artery and a vein. It is commonly associated with systemic telangiectasis, evident as red spots on the lips or mucous membranes. A large fistula may produce a murmur audible over the chest, but most often the lesion is silent. It is frequently asymptomatic, but the major clinical concern is hemoptysis, which may be sudden and quite large. The lesion is generally visible on the x-ray film of the chest. Suggestive features are the appearance of vessels leading in and out of a nodular or conglomerate lesion. Diagnosis is made by pulmonary angiography. Treatment of a single AV fistula is surgical resection.

Pulmonary AV fistulas may be multiple and there is an increased incidence of such lesions in cirrhosis of the liver. The reason for this is not clear, but there are sufficient AV communications in some patients to produce hypoxemia from right-to-left shunting. This is particularly true when the patient sits upright, probably because of distribution of more of the circulation to the dependent lung which contains more fistulas. This is in contrast to the usual finding of worsening hypoxemia in the supine position, particularly in cirrhosis with ascites, when the fluid in the abdomen compresses lung in the supine but not erect position.

NONCARDIOGENIC PULMONARY EDEMA

Most commonly the result of transudation of fluid from increased capillary pressure secondary to heart failure, pulmonary edema can also occur because of widespread capillary damage leading to increased permeability of capillaries with leakage of protein and edema fluid into the interstitium of the lung. In many cases, the capillary leakage may be so severe as to produce respiratory failure in the form of the adult respiratory distress syndrome, which will be considered in more detail in the next chapter. In other

Table 8–2   Some Causes of Noncardiac Pulmonary Edema

Drugs (narcotics, salicylates)
Pulmonary infection (influenza, tuberculosis)
Oxygen excess and oxygen lack (altitude)
Inhalation injury (aspiration, smoke)
Hematogenous injury (shock, trauma, sepsis, pancreatitis)
Sudden expansion of the lung
Pulmonary emboli
Neurogenic (head injury, seizures)
Transfusion and hemodialysis

instances, the pulmonary edema is transient and self-limited or responds promptly to treatment of the underlying disease.

Drugs

Pulmonary edema has been produced by a great many different drugs, particularly narcotics and even sedatives, which may act both by hypoxia and by direct action on pulmonary capillaries. Salicylate overdose has been associated with pulmonary edema, as has treatment with chlorothiazide and nitrogen mustards.

Infection

Pulmonary edema is a common feature of pulmonary infections. After all, the rapid migration of fluid through infected alveoli in lobar pneumococcal pneumonia is a form of localized pulmonary edema. Non-bacterial infection, notably primary influenza pneumonia, may be associated with rapidly progressive edema of both lungs, leading to adult respiratory distress syndrome (ARDS). Mycoplasmic pneumonia may present a similar pattern. Infection must always be considered as a cause of ARDS, and even acute tuberculosis has been reported as a potentially reversible cause of this dramatic condition.

Oxygen

Both oxygen excess and oxygen lack can cause pulmonary edema. Oxygen toxicity causes direct damage to pulmonary capillaries, and more than 40 per cent oxygen in inspired air may be associated with such a lesion. This is often hard to distinguish from the disease requiring oxygen therapy, but it is the reason for using only as much oxygen as absolutely necessary. Pulmonary edema also occurs in people who go to high altitudes, particularly people who have lived at a high altitude, gone to sea level, and then returned. The mechanism of this interesting response is unclear, but it is reasonable to ascend to high altitudes slowly, with ample time for acclimatization. It may be due to vasoconstriction of pulmonary capillaries, diverting the blood to smaller units of lung under excess pressure, which then leak fluid, or it may be due to leakage through the larger pulmonary arteries proximal to the vasoconstriction.

Injury

The pulmonary capillaries can be directly injured in a number of ways, and pulmonary edema follows aspiration either of large amounts of water, as in near drowning, or of gastric contents, as in Mendelson's syndrome. Inhalation of smoke may be followed by pulmonary edema, and there is often a latent period of more than 48 hours, which means that victims of smoke inhalation should be observed carefully to make sure that pulmonary edema does not develop after apparent recovery. Neither smoke inhalation nor aspiration should be treated prophylactically with antibiotics but, rather, one should wait for evidence of infection and recovery of the infecting organisms. There is no evidence that these or other forms of pulmonary edema can be prevented by corticosteroids. Pulmonary edema results from a wide variety of systemic disorders, including trauma. It may be associated with acute pancreatitis because of release of proteolytic enzymes into the blood stream, which reach and then damage the lung capillaries.

Unilateral

Unilateral pulmonary edema may follow rapid expansion of the lung after either thoracentesis or aspiration of air from a pneumothorax. The mechanism of this is not entirely clear, but it is most likely due to the fact that, when the lung is collapsed, the capillaries are not perfused with blood and become hypoxic. When the lung is suddenly expanded, the vulnerable capillaries become perfused and leak edematous fluid. It is for this reason that most clinicians advocate removal of no more than 1.5 liter of air or fluid at any one time.

Neurogenic

One of the most interesting forms of noncardiac pulmonary edema is that associated with lesions of the central nervous system. Experimentally, lesions in the region of the fourth ventricle produce very sudden pulmonary edema, which has been shown to be the result of systemic vasoconstriction with a sudden shift of blood into the lung causing the capillaries to become over-expanded and leak fluid. A similar reaction may occur in humans, and it is likely that the pulmonary edema that follows head injury, often occurring instantaneously, is the result of just such sudden shifts of blood into the lungs. The same mechanism may operate in the pulmonary edema that follows seizures, termed postictal edema, and in the rare case of pulmonary edema following the fainting lark and mess trick, a Valsalva maneuver performed during chest compression with sudden release. This may be one of the mechanisms for the pulmonary edema characteristic of shock lung, but this complex clinical problem is compounded by the effects of prolonged hypotension, fluid overload used in treatment, and products of proteolytic and hypoxic damage in organs of the body that have been traumatized.

Miscellaneous

Pulmonary emboli, either with blood clots or with fat after trauma, may be associated with pulmonary edema, and this is most likely the result of leakage of fluid from nonoccluded capillaries that have been overperfused because the rest of the circulation has been obstructed. Sepsis may be associated with widespread capillary damage, both in the lungs and elsewhere, with capillary leakage and edema. Uremia may produce pulmonary edema through a similar mechanism, and there have been reports of capillary leakage in the lung following treatment of diabetic ketoacidosis.

Pulmonary edema may be a form of transfusion reaction, apparently related to leukoagglutinins in the donor or recipient serum. Hemodialysis has been associated with reduction of circulating white blood cells and platelets, which apparently become sequestered in the lungs and may cause pulmonary edema.

This brief description of a wide variety of reactions associated with pulmonary edema emphasizes the vulnerability of the lung to a host of endogenous and exogenous insults. In most instances even severe edema is followed by complete recovery and one of the important points to keep in mind is to do no harm. Fluid overload in the treatment of shock may be a major contributor to some cases of shock lung; broad-spectrum prophylactic antibiotics after lung aspiration may lead to the development of an infection that is very difficult to treat; corticosteroids after aspiration of gastric contents have been associated with more impairment of lung function than no treatment at all. The possibility that pulmonary edema may occur when using a variety of drugs, blood transfusions, and oxygen and in performing procedures such as thoracentesis should be kept in mind.

Additional Reading

Heath D, Smith P: Pulmonary vascular disease. Med Clin North Am 61:1279–1308, 1977.
Moser KM: Pulmonary Embolism. Am Rev Respir Dis 115:829–852, 1977.
Reichel J: Pulmonary embolism. Med Clin North Am 61:1309–1318, 1977.
Shanies HM: Noncardiogenic pulmonary edema. Med Clin North Am 61:1319–1338, 1977.

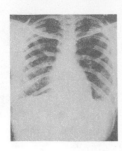

RESPIRATORY FAILURE

Respiratory failure is inability of the lungs to maintain normal arterial blood gas composition. After a review of the physiology involved in the maintenance of a normal arterial P_{CO_2} and P_{O_2} and the inter-relationships of P_{CO_2} with acidosis and alkalosis, the important causes of hypercapnia (ventilatory failure) will be discussed, with emphasis on the nature and extent of the abnormalities present in the various conditions that cause CO_2 retention. The primary physician is capable of managing many of these problems, but he must know when it is necessary to have the patient placed in a specialized respiratory care unit and when to consider intubation. Adult respiratory distress syndrome, an advanced form of noncardiac pulmonary edema, has become increasingly common in recent years, and it is the responsibility of the primary physician to make an early diagnosis and to hospitalize patients with the condition in a pulmonary intensive care unit.

PATHOPHYSIOLOGY

The principal function of the lungs is to maintain a normal arterial blood gas composition. Although hypercapnia is generally associated with some degree of hypoxemia, the converse is not true, and there are many patients with a reduced arterial oxygen tension in whom the arterial P_{CO_2} is normal or low. The practicing physician should understand the mechanisms responsible for hypercapnia and hypoxemia, and the circumstances under which they occur, so as to apply rational treatment.

Arterial Carbon Dioxide Tension (Paco₂)

The arterial P_{CO_2} is regulated by the alveolar ventilation and is the balance between the amount of air entering and leaving the alveoli each minute and the metabolic production of CO_2 by the tissues. Normally this balance is carefully regulated, and the arterial P_{CO_2} is kept constant at 40 mm Hg regardless of metabolic load. A sleeping person or a person heavily exercising, each with widely different metabolic productions of carbon dioxide, maintains the $Paco_2$ at 40 mm Hg. This integration is achieved by the respiratory center, which acts through the neuromuscular apparatus to produce an alveolar ventilation that is exactly appropriate to metabolic demand. Failure of this system requires relatively specific derangement and, in most instances, major degrees of abnormality. It should be recalled that the normal person is capable of a minute ventilation some 20 times the resting requirement, an indication of the enormous reserve of the respiratory system and the fact that severe disorder must be present before the Pco_2 rises.

The alveolar ventilation is not the same as the total ventilation, since some of the air entering and leaving the lung must pass in and out of the dead space. The physiological dead space is more than the volume of the tracheobronchial tree, since it includes units of lung that are ventilated but not perfused with blood. These units may become quite large in pulmonary disease, so that increase of the physiological dead space, as would occur in pulmonary embolism or other diseases in which there are units with a high ventilation/perfusion ratio, could lead to reduction of the alveolar ventilation despite a normal or increased total ventilation. In most instances, however, the increase of Pco_2 resulting from such ventilation/perfusion inequality stimulates the respiratory center to increase the total minute ventilation, keeping the arterial Pco_2 constant. In extreme disease, especially chronic obstructive pulmonary disease, the dead space may become so large because of the marked $\dot{V}/\dot{Q}$ inequalities that it contributes substantially to CO_2 retention, since there is a limited reserve for increasing the minute ventilation.

Hypocapnia

A reduced Pco_2 (hypocapnia) is always the result of excessive alveolar ventilation. It may result from anxiety or from a variety of diseases, such as diffuse interstitial disease or pulmonary embolism, which are associated with an increase of the reflex drive to breathe. It is poorly reflected in clinical signs and symptoms. Acute hyperventilation may be associated with so much respiratory alkalosis that dizziness and even syncope occur, but chronic hyperventilation is soon followed by bicarbonate excretion by the kidney, with return of pH towards normal.

Hypercapnia

Hypercapnia is also poorly reflected in symptomatology, though acute rise of Pco_2 is associated with respiratory distress from the increased drive to breathe. Chronic hypercapnia is associated with renal retention of bicarbonate, with restoration of Pco_2 towards normal and disappearance of symptoms. Increasing hypercapnia in a patient with chronic obstructive pulmonary disease may be associated with somnolence and, ultimately, a decreased ventilatory drive, but accurate assessment of the alveolar ventilation requires measurement of the arterial Pco_2.

Alteration of the Pco_2 is important because of associated changes of pH (Fig. 9–1). Hypocapnia causes alkalosis, and hypercapnia causes acidosis. These changes are ultimately buffered by appropriate changes of serum

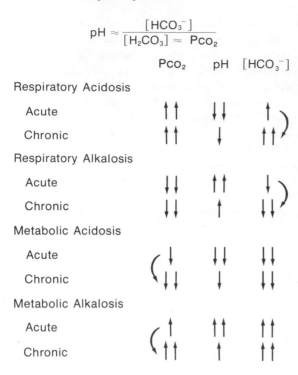

$$pH \approx \frac{[HCO_3^-]}{[H_2CO_3]} \approx P_{CO_2}$$

	P_{CO_2}	pH	$[HCO_3^-]$
Respiratory Acidosis			
Acute	↑↑	↓↓	↑
Chronic	↑↑	↓	↑↑
Respiratory Alkalosis			
Acute	↓↓	↑↑	↓
Chronic	↓↓	↑	↓↓
Metabolic Acidosis			
Acute	↓	↓↓	↓↓
Chronic	↓↓	↓	↓↓
Metabolic Alkalosis			
Acute	↑	↑↑	↑↑
Chronic	↑↑	↑	↑↑

Figure 9–1 Respiratory and metabolic acidosis and alkalosis. The pH is proportional to the ratio $\frac{HCO_3^-}{H_2CO_3}$. H_2CO_3 is directly proportional to P_{CO_2}. Respiratory acidosis is due to increased P_{CO_2} and if this is sustained, renal retention of bicarbonate causes pH to return towards normal. Acute respiratory alkalosis is due to reduction of P_{CO_2} (carbonic acid), which is followed by renal excretion of bicarbonate with return of pH towards normal.

Metabolic acidosis is due to reduction of bicarbonate because of the production of stronger acids. This is followed by hyperventilation so that P_{CO_2} falls with return of pH towards normal. Metabolic alkalosis is due to a primary increase of serum bicarbonate followed by hypoventilation with a rise of P_{CO_2} and a return of pH towards normal.

bicarbonate induced by renal excretion and retention, respectively. It is occasionally difficult to distinguish between respiratory and metabolic acidosis and alkalosis. Respiratory acidosis results from increased P_{CO_2}, and a low pH in association with hypercapnia can be attributed to decreased alveolar ventilation. Not uncommonly, however, acute respiratory failure, as in severe asthma, is associated with decreased cardiac output or sufficient arterial oxygen unsaturation to cause severe hypoxemia with lactic acidosis. There is, then, an added metabolic component to the acidosis, which can only be assessed if the physician is familiar with the expected changes of pH in association with uncomplicated CO_2 retention. As a rule of thumb, acute increase of P_{CO_2} of 10 mm Hg is associated with 0.10 unit decrease of pH. If the pH is decreased more than expected from the rise of P_{CO_2}, metabolic acidosis complicates the respiratory acidosis.

Bicarbonate retention is the physiologic compensation for respiratory acidosis. It is the primary abnormality in metabolic alkalosis associated with potassium or chloride deficiency. Such electrolyte abnormalities are not uncommon in patients with COPD, particularly when treated with diuretics. As with acidosis, the respiratory and metabolic components of the increase $[HCO_3]$ can be assessed and sorted out from knowledge of how much the serum bicarbonate should rise for a given increase of P_{CO_2}. If the bicarbonate is higher than expected for the degree of CO_2 retention, metabolic alkalosis complicates the chronic respiratory acidosis. If the blood is alkaline, or even if the pH is normal in the presence of increased P_{CO_2}, one must suspect the presence of metabolic alkalosis in addition to the compensated respiratory acidosis.

Respiratory alkalosis and metabolic acidosis are both associated with a reduced P_{CO_2}, but the pH is high in the former, low in the latter. In the compensated state, pH is returned toward normal. Metabolic acidosis is compensated by hyperventilation, leading to decreased P_{CO_2} and $[H_2CO_3]$, but the blood remains slightly acidic. Respiratory alkalosis, for which compensation is achieved by renal excretion of bicarbonate so as to restore pH towards normal, is associated with slight alkalinity of the blood.

Arterial Oxygen Tension (Pao₂)

The arterial oxygen tension is also regulated by the alveolar ventilation, but it is much more sensitive to other disturbances of pulmonary function. Changes of ventilation alone will cause about as much change of arterial P_{O_2} as of P_{CO_2}, but it should be recalled that increase of arterial P_{O_2} is without consequence, whereas a decreased P_{CO_2} causes alkalosis. Decrease of arterial P_{O_2} has to be substantial, because of the flat upper portion of the oxygen dissociation curve, before significant hypoxemia develops. Thus, the alveolar ventilation is primarily important in regulating P_{CO_2}, and only extreme hypoventilation will be associated with significant hypoxemia.

However, the arterial P_{O_2} is much more sensitive to alterations of diffusion, circulation, and ventilation/perfusion homogeneity in the lung. Oxygen is so much less diffusible than carbon dioxide that marked reduction of the diffusion capacity can cause reduction of arterial P_{O_2} without any change in the P_{CO_2}. In fact, however, the diffusing capacity must be extremely low, less than 25 per cent of normal, before significant hypoxemia occurs, and arterial unsaturation is practically never the result of impaired diffusion alone. If the diffusing capacity is very low, the increased demands for oxygen uptake imposed by exercise may be associated with a significant fall of arterial oxygen tension and saturation, and this may contribute to dyspnea and even to polycythemia in some patients with advanced interstitial disease of the lung.

Right-to-left shunts also are associated with hypoxemia. The reason that hypoxemia is more significant than hypercapnia is that the venous oxygen tension is much lower than the arterial oxygen tension, whereas the venous carbon dioxide tension is only a little higher than the arterial P_{CO_2}. Thus, when venous blood mixes with arterialized blood in the lung because of a right-to-left shunt there is much more effect on the arterial oxygen tension and saturation than on the arterial P_{CO_2}. Furthermore, an increase of P_{CO_2} is associated with hyperventilation to return the P_{CO_2} to normal, but this will fail to compensate for the hypoxemia.

The most common and important cause of hypoxemia in pulmonary disease is ventilation/perfusion inequality in the lung. Units overperfused with respect to ventilation contain a P_{O_2} that is much lower than normal and will contribute to arterial unsaturation. These units will also contain a high P_{CO_2}; but other units, which are overventilated relative to perfusion, will contain a much lower P_{CO_2} and tend to compensate for the derangement. No such compensation is available for oxygen because the normal $\dot{V}/\dot{Q}$ ratio provides practically full oxygenation of the blood; and, again because of the flat upper portion of the oxygen dissociation curve, hyperventilation cannot increase arterial oxygen saturation further so as to compensate for the low $\dot{V}/\dot{Q}$ units. Furthermore any increase of PCO_2 will be associated with hyperventilation, which will correct the carbon dioxide retention but not the hypoxemia. $\dot{V}/\dot{Q}$ abnormalities can occur in a wide variety of diseases and are the major cause of hypoxemia in obstructive lung disease, diffuse interstitial disease of the lung, and pulmonary edema.

Signs and symptoms of hypoxemia are just as unreliable as those of hypercapnia. Acute hypoxia may be associated with some alteration of mental status and blurring of consciousness, but this often takes the form of euphoria, so that it is not unpleasant and not associated with respiratory distress. The hyperventilation induced by hypoxemia, unlike that associated with acute hypercapnia, is relatively mild and may not cause noticeable dyspnea. Likewise, the signs of hypoxemia are unreliable, and severe arterial unsaturation must be present before the physician can detect cyanosis. Furthermore, cyanosis is importantly modified by other factors, including skin capillarity and the concentration of hemoglobin in the blood. It may be evident in the extremities or lips because of local vasoconstriction, as in cold weather. Thus, significant hypoxemia can occur without detectable cyanosis, and cyanosis may be present when the arterial oxygen saturation is normal. It is imperative to obtain measurements of arterial blood gas composition if there is any reason to suspect either hypercapnia or hypoxemia.

ADAPTATIONS TO HYPOXIA

There are very important mechanisms that operate to compensate for chronic hypoxemia, and they are best illustrated by exposure to increased altitude. Rapid ascent to a higher altitude leads, acutely, to hyperventilation. The resultant alkalosis accounts for the symptoms of nausea, vomiting, and even Cheyne-Stokes respiration at night that characterize acute mountain sickness. These symptoms disappear when renal excretion of bicarbonate restores the pH to normal, thus permitting maintenance of the hyperventilation without alkalosis.

Like continued residence at high altitudes, chronic hypoxemia because of lung disease leads to a number of adaptations that permit continuation of life and even health. The reduced arterial PO_2 causes increased ventilation and, in addition, stimulates formation of erythropoietin, causing increased erythropoiesis. The increased hematocrit serves to bring more oxygen to the tissues. There is also increase of the cardiac output. Most importantly, there is expansion of the capillary bed in various organs of the body so that the oxygen-carrying red blood cells are brought closer to the intracellular mitochondria, which are the ultimate consumers of oxygen. This increased diffusibility of oxygen into the tissues is the most important adjustment to hypoxia and permits individuals with chronic hypoxemia to function normally in the face of arterial oxygen tensions that are so low as to be fatal to the unacclimatized subject. Patients can enter the hospital fully alert and functional with an arterial PO_2 as low as 20 mm Hg, or a mountaineer can climb to great heights with an arterial PO_2 as low as 40 mm Hg, levels that are associated with death and unconsciousness, respectively, in the unacclimatized subject.

Some of the compensations, however, are not beneficial. Pulmonary vasoconstriction in response to hypoxemia seems to serve little purpose but does cause pulmonary hypertension and, ultimately, right heart failure with venous congestion. It is known that salt and water retention and systemic venous congestion in chronic obstructive pulmonary disease are largely reversible by correcting arterial blood gas tensions and are more the result of acidosis and hypoxemia than failure of the right ventricle itself.

OXYGEN THERAPY

Most types of hypoxemia are successfully treated by increasing the inspired oxygen concentration. The only exception to this is right-to-left shunting, under which circumstance the arterial Po_2 only rises a little bit when extra oxygen is added to the inspired air. This is the basis for calculating the magnitude of right-to-left shunts, since any hypoxemia present during pure oxygen breathing can be attributed to shunting. Even when $\dot{V}/\dot{Q}$ disturbances are profound, adding oxygen to the inspired air causes elevation of the oxygen tension in the very poorly ventilated alveoli, with substantial improvement of arterial Po_2.

Oxygen can be administered in many ways. A loose-fitting Venturi mask exposes the patient to a constant atmosphere of oxygen of known composition. This is a relatively comfortable, precise way of administering oxygen, and it is particularly suitable for the very hypoxemic patient, in whom small changes of inspired oxygen may lead to hypoventilation. By using increasing concentrations of oxygen with different masks, one can gradually raise the arterial Po_2 while, at the same time, making certain that the arterial Pco_2 fails to rise further. Some patients fail to tolerate a Venturi mask, and it is perfectly acceptable to administer oxygen by nasal prongs, gradually increasing the flow rate of oxygen to the nasal passages as dictated by the changes in arterial blood gas composition. In patients on respirators, the inspired oxygen concentration can, of course, be regulated precisely.

It is now possible to provide chronic oxygen therapy for the outpatient. Oxygen tanks can be the source of oxygen by either Venturi mask or nasal prongs, and portable tanks of liquid oxygen are light enough for the ambulatory patient to continue to receive the treatment. The indications for this type of therapy are not entirely clear, since the adjustments to chronic hypoxemia may be so effective as to make chronic oxygen therapy unnecessary. In some patients oxygen may improve exercise tolerance. It may reduce pulmonary hypertension and prevent right heart failure. If secondary polycythemia is deleterious because of increased viscosity of the blood, it may reduce the need for phlebotomy. There is recent evidence that it actually prolongs life, and long-term trials now under way should provide better guidance about the indications for this type of treatment.

VENTILATORY FAILURE

Fairly specific and generally very extensive abnormalities of the integrated system responsible for maintenance of minute ventilation must be present

Table 9–1   Causes of Ventilatory Failure

Central Nervous System
    Drugs
    Infections
    Trauma
    Primary alveolar hypoventilation
Neuromuscular
    Infection
    Neuromuscular blockade
    Trauma
    Neuromyopathy
Chest Cage
    Kyphoscoliosis
    Obesity
    Trauma
    Pleural effusion and fibrosis
Metabolic
    Hypokalemia
    Hypophosphatemia
    Alkalosis
    Myxedema
Restrictive Lung Disease
Obstructive Lung Disease
Upper Airway Obstruction

before the system fails and CO_2 retention develops. The rate and depth of respiration are precisely regulated by the respiratory center, acting through the motor nerves to the muscles of the chest wall and diaphragm to inflate and deflate the lungs. The latter must be relatively compliant and unobstructed for ventilation to proceed with ease. It is appropriate to review the disturbances that occur at each of these levels so as to understand in what kinds of patients hypoventilation may occur and how it can best be corrected.

The major therapeutic problem in patients with ventilatory failure is maintenance of adequate ventilation, and the indication for artificial ventilation varies with the underlying cause and the acuteness of the problem. In addition, there is a variable degree of hypoxemia, depending upon the nature of the underlying disease. In individuals with normal lungs in whom hypoventilation is largely a result of neuromuscular disease, hypoxemia may be a mild problem, though usually the subnormal ventilation is associated with some degree of atelectasis and right-to-left shunting with hypoxemia. This can be minimized by periodic inflation of the lung with deep breaths as a substitute for the normal signs and yawns. By widely opening all alveolar units, deep breaths reverse the subclinical atelectasis, which is otherwise apt to develop during prolonged quiet breathing. In patients with lung disease responsible for ventilatory failure, hypoxemia is usually the dominant problem, and when respiratory infection complicates neuromuscular disease, the same may be true. This will require appropriate therapy with oxygen.

Central Nervous System

Located in the brain stem, the respiratory center is endowed with intrinsic automaticity and with such an extensive blood supply that it is relatively invulnerable to extensive disease of the central nervous system. Thus, extensive brain damage from hypoxia, drugs, or cerebral vascular disease may produce total loss of cerebral cortical function without interfering with automatic respiration. One does not expect ventilatory failure to result from a cerebral vascular accident.

Drugs

After acute drug intoxication or other insults, respiratory periodicity will generally remain even though cerebral function is lost. On the other hand, some types of drug overdose may produce so much depression of the respiratory neurons that hypoventilation results. This is particularly the case with narcotics, which act on the respiratory centers, and heroin and methadone overdose are much more commonly associated with hypoventilation than is overdose with barbiturates.

It should be recalled that surgery can be performed under barbiturate anesthesia without the need for ventilatory support. Although intubation is generally advised for patients with acute drug overdose, in order to maintain a patent airway, artificial ventilation is not always needed and should be employed as indicated by measurements of arterial carbon dioxide tension. Administration of the appropriate antagonist, such as naloxone for heroin overdose, may lead to such prompt arousal as to obviate the need for intubation at all.

Infection

Specific infections of the central nervous system, notably poliomyelitis and some forms of viral encephalitis, may affect the respiratory centers enough to produce hypoventilation and, ultimately, the need for respiratory support. As in many other conditions, this is generally reflected in profound paralysis, but it is important to assess ventilatory function by measuring vital capacity in patients with such conditions so as to recognize the development of respiratory muscle dysfunction and to be prepared to institute artificial ventilation if the P_{CO_2} rises.

Trauma

Trauma to the brain stem may be associated with hypoventilation because of injury to the respiratory center, and surgical treatment of intractable pain by percutaneous cordotomy of the spinal-thalamic tracts in the upper cervical region has been associated with temporary loss of automatic ventilation because of interruption of afferent impulses to the respiratory center. Patients who have undergone this procedure must be watched carefully, particularly when they fall asleep, to make certain that they continue to breathe with normal regularity.

Primary Alveolar Hypoventilation

Primary alveolar hypoventilation is a rare disorder of great physiological interest because it is apparently a unique, localized disturbance of the respiratory center, perhaps the result of viral encephalitis, in which there is loss of the normal sensitivity to carbon dioxide. Patients with this syndrome have totally normal heart and lungs and are able to breathe normally with normal lung volumes on command, but they fail to maintain normal respiratory periodicity and, as a result, experience chronic hypercapnia. Their respiration is characteristically irregular, with more hypoventilation during sleep than wakefulness, and a diagnostic finding is total lack of sensitivity to inhalation of increased concentrations of carbon dioxide. Patients with other types of impairment of the respiratory system may not respond with a normal increase of ventilation when they breathe carbon dioxide because there is so much mechanical interference to the act of respiration. These patients do have some response, however, in contrast to the absence of any response at all in the primary alveolar hypoventilation syndrome.

It is interesting that these patients do not complain of respiratory symptoms, since they have no respiratory distress and are unaware of the underlying problem. Their symptoms result from chronic hypercapnia and hypoxemia. Most of them present with systemic circulatory congestion: elevation of venous pressure, enlargement of the right ventricle, and edema. The diagnosis can be suspected when a patient presents with right heart failure for no apparent reason in association with elevated arterial P_{CO_2}. The finding of normal lungs on x-ray examination and physiological study is strong evidence that the condition exists, but a CO_2 response should be measured for absolute confirmation of the diagnosis. These patients can be taught to breathe normally when awake, but they generally hypoventilate during sleep, when they are particularly liable to increasing and fatal hypoventilation unless given ventilatory support, as in a tank respirator or with a body cuirass. A unique therapy is now available by which the implantation of electrodes on the phrenic nerves makes it possible to pace the diaphragm and induce normal rhythmic respiration, just as one paces the heart when its conduction system is deranged.

Neuromuscular

Because of the extensive reserve, widespread involvement of the neuromuscular system must be present before ventilation becomes inadequate.

Guillain-Barré Syndrome

Peripheral neuropathy, once most commonly the result of poliomyelitis, is now most often the result of Guillain-Barré syndrome. This syndrome may evolve with devastating speed, leading to total respiratory paralysis within a few hours of the onset of symptoms. Patients with this disease must be watched very carefully with serial measurements of vital capacity in order to detect respiratory muscle weakness. Most physicians now feel that if the vital capacity falls to 1 liter, particularly at a rapid rate, artificial ventilation should be instituted.

Neuromuscular Blockade

Neuromuscular blockade can be produced by the injection of curariform drugs, by the administration of some antibiotics such as the aminoglycosides, by botulin toxin, and by myasthenia gravis. In all of these conditions, as in the Guillain-Barré syndrome, the respiratory paralysis may proceed with extreme rapidity, so that the appropriate diagnosis is extremely important. In puzzling cases of ventilatory failure, a tensilon test may be of diagnostic value. In most cases ventilatory support is easily maintained with a respirator until the cause of the neuromuscular blockade has disappeared or until effective treatment of myasthenia has been instituted with cholinergic drugs or ACTH. It is noteworthy that appropriate respiratory care has made thymectomy so much more feasible that it has become a common treatment for myasthenia gravis.

High Cervical Trauma

High cervical trauma interferes with neuromuscular function only if there is interference with the function of the phrenic nerves, since the diaphragm alone is more than capable of sustaining ventilatory function. In such cases, diaphragmatic pacing may be effective.

Neuromuscular Disease

Neuromuscular disease must be extremely advanced before the respiratory muscles fail. Ventilatory failure has been described in tetanus and may be a complication of spinal cord disease, such as multiple sclerosis, or of extensive muscular dystrophy. In the latter conditions, liability to respiratory infection because of inadequate cough and the tendency to aspirate is apt to cause more of a problem than is chronic hypoventilation; it is very rare for multiple sclerosis actually to cause ventilatory failure. Patients with muscular dystrophy may have profound respiratory paralysis, with a vital capacity as low as 600 cc, and yet maintain adequate alveolar ventilation. They may, however, require respiratory support during intercurrent infections and ultimately require chronic therapy with a respirator. As in other diseases affecting the neuromuscular regulation of respiration, artificial ventilation is easily achieved because lung and chest mechanics are normal, and a cuirass respirator may be a practical solution and avoids the need for intubation or chronic tracheostomy.

Chest Cage

Kyphoscoliosis

As emphasized in Chapter 7, *kyphoscoliosis* may be associated with obvious and marked spinal deformity without causing hypoventilation, and most patients are able to continue to function even though the vital capacity may be far less than 1 liter. Episodic worsening, often related to respiratory infection, may require intensive care and even intubation with a short period of artificial ventilation. The value of periodic inflation of the lungs with IPPB was described previously.

Obesity

Obesity is commonly associated with hypoventilation, and the mechanisms of this interesting phenomenon have been described in Chapter 6, with emphasis on the importance of the associated airway obstruction, which is often present during sleep in these patients.

Trauma

Chest trauma is rarely associated with hypoventilation unless there is bilateral injury with flail chest, under which circumstances intubation and artificial ventilation may be necessary. Injury to the diaphragm is usually not associated with hypoventilation, but bilateral diaphragmatic paralysis may be accompanied by CO_2 retention in the supine position, when the weight of the abdominal contents causes elevation of the diaphragm and further impairment of lung function.

Pleural Disease

It is only the rare case of very extensive pleural disease, large bilateral pleural effusions, or extensive scarring of both pleural surfaces that leads to hypoventilation, and most patients can tolerate marked restriction of lung movement without developing CO_2 retention.

Metabolic

There are a number of metabolic derangements that may be associated with so much respiratory muscle weakness as to cause hypoventilation.

Electrolyte Imbalance

Hypokalemia may be so profound as to produce muscle paralysis, including the muscles of respiration, as may hypophosphatemia, which is becoming increasingly recognized as an acute metabolic consequence of a variety of disorders.

Alkalosis

Hypoventilation is the appropriate physiological compensation for alkalosis, and it is wrong to administer artificial ventilation to a patient whose chronic elevation of bicarbonate is appropriately compensated by CO_2 retention induced by reduction of alveolar ventilation. Generally alkalosis is associated with only mild degrees of hypoventilation, and the Pco_2 is rarely higher than 50 mm Hg, though substantially higher values have been described in severe cases. Treatment must be directed at the underlying metabolic abnormality; and as the serum bicarbonate falls, the ventilation will return to normal. In some patients with chronic obstructive pulmonary disease the administration of diuretics may be associated with chloride depletion and alkalosis out of proportion to the required compensation. This may make it difficult to restore the Pco_2 to normal, since reduction of Pco_2 will now be associated with rise of pH and feedback inhibition of ventilation. Chloride replacement, usually with potassium chloride, may correct the metabolic alkalosis and make it possible for the alveolar ventilation to increase as the obstructive pulmonary disease abates.

Hypothyroidism

In some cases severe hypothyroidism may be associated with hypoventilation, and one cause of death from myxedema coma has been ventilatory failure. The mechanism for this is not entirely clear, but there is evidence that the hypoventilation is the result of a decrease of muscle strength. It is important to recognize this possibility, to test ventilatory function by measurement of vital capacity, and to be ready to employ artificial ventilation if CO_2 retention develops. Patients with severe myxedema may respond quite slowly to thyroid therapy, and it is wise to maintain ventilatory support, or at least to keep the patient under careful observation in an intensive care unit, until there is clear evidence of return of thyroid function towards normal.

Restrictive Lung Disease

As emphasized in Chapter 5, diffuse lung disease is rarely so extensive as to cause hypoventilation. In fact, the associated increase of the reflex drive to breathe generally produces hyperventilation. In very advanced cases, particularly if associated with other derangement, hypercapnia may develop and require ventilatory support. Acute respiratory failure in association with diffuse lung injury is discussed under Adult Respiratory Distress Syndrome.

Obstructive Lung Disease

By far the most common cause of hypercapnia is obstructive lung disease, outnumbering all the other causes together manyfold. As emphasized in Chapter 2, ventilatory failure may occur in very severe asthma, but the vast majority of patients with asthma have a lower than normal Pco_2 because of the extra stimuli to ventilation that are present. When the obstruction becomes overwhelming, the Pco_2 may rise, and the patient requires careful observation in an intensive care unit for the indications for intubation and artificial ventilation outlined in Chapter 2. Hypercapnia is much more common in chronic obstructive pulmonary disease (COPD), perhaps because the disease is chronic and not associated with the acute stimulation to ventilation so common in asthma.

There is considerable variation, but most people with hypercapnia due to COPD have an FEV_1 below 1 liter and an FEV25-75% less than 0.5 l/sec. Considerable obstruction, particularly in patients with emphysema ("pink puffers") may be present without CO_2 retention, and there are patients with an FEV25-75% as low as 0.3 l/sec who maintain their Pco_2 in the low 30's. Many patients with COPD have chronic hypercapnia all the time, and the measures used in the treatment of this condition have been outlined in Chapter 3. Acute ventilatory failure, or an acute increase of the chronically elevated Pco_2, requires special attention and careful treatment in a respiratory intensive care unit. It is usually the result of some increase of the chronically elevated airway resistance and often the result of respiratory infection and the associated increase of secretions, which are imperfectly cleared from the tracheobronchial tree. The injudicious use of tranquilizers and sedatives may potentiate this development, and these drugs should be avoided when possible in COPD, certainly during any exacerbation.

Treatment

The treatment of ventilatory failure due to COPD requires careful attention and judgment. Immediate therapy includes the measures outlined in Chapter 3: antibiotics for associated infection, hydration, bronchodilators, and physical measures designed to induce deep breathing and effective cough. Arterial blood gas composition must be measured promptly, and if the arterial oxygen saturation is significantly reduced, the patient should be given inspired oxygen in low concentration either by Venturi mask or by nasal prongs. This must be followed by another measurement of arterial Pco_2, since elimination of the extra hypoxic drive to breathe may be sufficient to cause further hypoventilation, with a dangerous rise of Pco_2 and fall of pH. It is for this reason that oxygen is given in slowly increasing concentrations, with careful monitoring of the effect on the arterial blood gases.

The indications for intubation in COPD require the same kind of judgment as in asthma. As long as the patient can cooperate with therapy by coughing, raising secretions, and taking deep breaths, there is probably no set level of Pco_2 that mandates intubation. If the patient becomes seriously obtunded, artificial ventilation may be necessary and, then, ventilation should be administered in conjunction with serial measurements of arterial Pco_2 and pH. The inspired oxygen concentration is kept at the level needed to maintain a normal arterial Po_2.

It is important to remember that patients with ventilatory failure secondary to COPD generally have chronic hypercapnia with substantial bicarbonate retention, and the ventilation should be adjusted to bring the Pco_2 down only to a level that is associated with a normal or only slightly alkaline pH. Later, as bicarbonate is excreted by the kidney, the ventilation can be increased until the Pco_2 is brought down to a normal level. Many patients with COPD and chronic CO_2 retention are unable to maintain a normal arterial Pco_2, and in that case the Pco_2 should be lowered only to the level at which it had been maintained in the chronic state. If the Pco_2 is brought to normal, the associated bicarbonate excretion will mean that when the patient is taken off the respirator and cannot maintain the Pco_2 at that level, the resultant acute acidosis will be intolerable, and it will be impossible to wean the patient from the respirator.

Patients with ventilatory failure due to COPD are notably at risk of developing pulmonary emboli and gastrointestinal bleeding. Therapy should include prophylactic administration of antacids and, probably, small doses of heparin to prevent phlebothrombosis. To prevent gastrointestinal bleeding, antacids should be given in a dose sufficient to maintain the gastric pH over 3.5. This requires nasogastric intubation, which is probably not warranted unless the patient is seriously ill or on a respirator and requires a nasogastric tube anyway. There are some who believe that corticosteroids are of value, but the evidence for this is not convincing. If there is indication of an asthmatic component to the obstruction, and if the sputum contains eosinophils on Wright's stain, steroids may be used.

It is important to pay particular attention to fluid and electrolyte balance in these patients. Hypokalemia and hypophosphatemia may contribute to respiratory muscle weakness, and metabolic alkalosis from excessive diuretics may make it difficult to restore ventilation to the chronic level.

Various respiratory stimulants have been advocated for patients with hypercapnia, particularly that developing during oxygen therapy and indicating a potential for reversibility. There are conflicting data about the value of aminophylline in this situation, and other drugs such as nikethamide and benzedrine have been associated with increased ventilation in conjunction with general cortical stimulation. In patients with chronic CO_2 retention, these respiratory stimulants probably have little role, since effective action is often associated with significant sleep deprivation. On the other hand, progesterone has been used with good effect in a number of patients with hypercapnia due to chronic lung disease, and it seems to be particularly useful in obesity. Some patients with chronic obstructive pulmonary disease have also responded to this therapy.

Upper Airway Obstruction

Sleep apnea resulting from upper airway obstruction, a notable feature of the Pickwickian syndrome, has been described in Chapter 7. Chronic upper airway obstruction may also result from tracheal stenosis, a not uncommon complication of intubation, from vocal cord paralysis, or from compression of the trachea by a large goiter or tumor. The diagnosis should be suspected when dyspnea is associated with inspiratory and expiratory stridor, but it may be necessary to have the patient breathe deeply in order to reveal this sign. In uncertain cases, the diagnosis can be made with confidence by measuring inspiratory and expiratory flow rates. In obstructive pulmonary disease, interference with flow rates is primarily evident during expiration, and inspiration is relatively normal and unimpeded. In contrast, when the obstruction is due to fixed narrowing of the trachea or even the large bronchi, interference with flow rates is equally present during inspiration and expiration, so that there is reduction of inspiratory as well as expiratory flow rates. It is important to bear this possibility in mind, and, if there is any question about the cause of airway obstruction, to make the appropriate measurement so as to be able to provide specific surgical therapy.

Upper airway obstruction is particularly dangerous because it may lead to serious degrees of hypercapnia without as much dyspnea as commonly present in patients with obstructive lung disease, perhaps because the inspiratory obstruction, which is the main cause of hypoventilation, is not associated with as much respiratory distress as is severe expiratory obstruction. As a guide, if the flow rate during the middle half of inspiration is less than 1 liter per second, severe, fixed obstruction of the airways is present and the patient should be put under immediate observation with a view to surgical correction.

ADULT RESPIRATORY DISTRESS SYNDROME (ARDS)

Acute failure of the oxygenation function of the lungs may occur without significant CO_2 retention. The wide variety of patients in which this occurs has been described in Chapter 8 (Noncardiac Pulmonary Edema). The common denominator of the condition is excessive transudation of fluid through pulmonary capillaries, sometimes because of increased permeability from a variety of causes and sometimes because of sudden overexpansion of the capillary bed with resultant leakage of protein-containing fluid. In the early stages, just as in cardiac pulmonary edema, the fluid passes from the capillaries into the interstitium of the lung and tracks up along perivascular and peribronchial sheaths. The first physiological evidence of abnormality is revealed by sensitive tests of small airway function. The roentgenogram may only reveal some increased vascular markings and redistribution of the circulation from the lower to the upper portions of the lung, with characteristic fuzzy enlargement of the pulmonary vessels in the upper lobes. Later, the fluid is spilled over into the alveoli, with encroachment upon the gas-exchanging air spaces. At this stage the lungs become very stiff, and the fluid-filled alveolar units perfused with blood cause a right-to-left shunt, which may be extensive and may cause severe hypoxemia. At this stage the roentgenogram reveals diffuse increase of alveolar densities, generally with an air bronchogram.

In individuals at risk, such as those who have suffered traumatic shock or undergone extensive surgery, victims of heroin or methadone overdose, patients with primary influenza pneumonia, and the many others listed in Chapter 8, ARDS should be suspected at the first sign of respiratory distress, which is usually an increase in respiratory rate. Because of the vascular congestion, there is reflex stimulation to ventilation and the arterial P_{CO_2} is characteristically reduced. The earliest simple test suggesting the development of pulmonary edema is measurement of the arterial oxygen tension, with demonstration of a widening of the alveolar-arterial oxygen gradient. Just as in pulmonary embolism, the arterial P_{O_2} may be near normal because of the marked hyperventilation and increase of the alveolar oxygen tension. But the A-a gradient, indicative of the $\dot{V}/\dot{Q}$ abnormalities present in the congested lung, is widened.

Management

Management, in addition to treatment of the underlying condition, is directed at maintaining oxygenation. Increasing concentrations of inspired oxygen should be used as needed to maintain the arterial oxygen tension around 70 mm Hg. Patients requiring such treatment should be managed in a respiratory care unit with skilled inhalation therapy and physiological monitoring. If the arterial oxygen cannot be maintained at a satisfactory level with inspired oxygen concentrations of 40 per cent or higher or if there is increasing evidence of fatigue and respiratory distress, intubation may be indicated in order to apply positive end-expiratory pressure (PEEP). It has been shown that this treatment maintains expansion of the lung at the end of expiration, so that the edematous alveolar units are kept open rather than collapsing and causing increasing shunting. It has further been shown that such treatment can maintain the arterial Po_2 at a satisfactory level without the need for potentially dangerous concentrations of inspired oxygen. The evidence that such treatment actually has beneficial effects in decreasing the formation of edematous fluid in the lungs is contradictory. In any event, careful management of the ventilation to maintain optimal arterial Po_2 without causing reduction of cardiac output by increasing intrathoracic pressure too much is essential.

Other measures, such as corticosteroids and plasma expanders, have not proven to be of value in ARDS of a variety of etiologies, though there is some evidence that a minimal capillary fluid volume tends to reduce edema formation. However, it is necessary to maintain systemic blood pressure, and diuretic therapy should be guided by measurement of intravascular pressures, including the wedge pressure. Patients requiring this type of management have an extremely high mortality.

Although ARDS is primarily a failure of oxygenation, in late stages the lungs may become so overloaded with fluid as to be unable to exchange carbon dioxide properly, and arterial Pco_2 may rise. This usually can be satisfactorily treated with the artificial respiration used in conjunction with administration of PEEP.

In patients in whom maximal ventilatory support fails to produce adequate oxygenation, tissue oxygen supply can be maintained by extracorporeal perfusion through a membrane oxygenator. Attempts have been made to improve the very poor survival rate that is present in this condition with this type of therapy, but the results have not been sufficiently good to warrant continuing use of the procedure except as an experimental measure.

Some patients with overwhelming respiratory failure from ARDS have survived, even after prolonged therapy with artificial ventilation. In many such patients, pulmonary function has returned to normal, even though lung biopsy revealed what appeared to be diffuse fibrosis during the acute illness. For that reason it is very worthwhile to maintain maximum therapeutic efforts, regardless of the apparent extent of lung damage, in the hope that there will be full recovery.

The main concern of the primary physician is to have knowledge of the many conditions that can cause ARDS, to attempt to prevent it, and to recognize its development at an early stage so that the patient can be placed in an appropriate intensive respiratory care unit for continuing management.

Additional Reading

Martin L: Respiratory Failure. Med Clin North Am 61:1397–1408, 1977.

Pierce AK: Acute respiratory failure. In Gunter CA, Welch MH, (eds): Pulmonary Medicine. Philadelphia, J. B. Lippincott, 1977.

Pontoppidan H, Geffin B, Lowenstein E: Acute respiratory failure in the adult. N Engl J Med 287:690–698, 743–752, 799–806, 1972.

Williams MH Jr, Shim CS: Ventilatory failure. Am J Med 48:477–483, 1970.

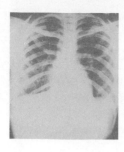

CHAPTER TEN

RESPIRATORY EMERGENCIES

True respiratory emergencies are quite rare, but the life or death outcome is so dependent upon proper recognition and management that the practicing physician must be prepared to cope with them. In many of the diseases considered previously, such as pulmonary infections, prompt diagnosis and treatment are essential, but generally there is time to obtain data and to formulate a therapeutic plan. This final chapter will deal with some problems for which immediate action is essential and with some other life-threatening pulmonary emergencies that require prompt, appropriate action. Severe chest trauma, which always presents multiple problems, must be managed by a team, including anesthesiologist and thoracic surgeon, and will not be considered.

APNEA

Respiratory arrest is the end result of ventilatory failure, which was considered in the previous chapter. However, there are some conditions in which progression to apnea may occur with extraordinary rapidity, and these require special emphasis.

Clearly the first priority is to establish adequate ventilation and to evaluate heart beat so as to restore circulation by closed-chest massage if indicated. After determining patency of the airway, artificial respiration can be maintained by mouth-to-mouth breathing, followed, as soon as possible, by insertion of an endotracheal tube and ventilation with a respirator. In performing mouth-to-mouth respiration, one must remember to extend the neck in order to prevent occlusion of the pharynx by the tongue, and to close the nostrils so that the lungs are properly ventilated.

Respiratory arrest is commonly associated with *cardiac arrest*, as after myocardial infarction, and resuscitation requires both closed-chest cardiac massage and artificial ventilation. It may also develop in the patients with the many types of *ventilatory failure* described in the previous chapter. But it may also be the presenting problem in a number of specific conditions.

Neuromuscular Paralysis

Rapidly progressive neuromuscular paralysis may lead to respiratory arrest before adequate recognition by either the patient or the physician. The Guillain-Barré syndrome, botulism, and myasthenia may also progress with such rapidity that the physician must be mindful of these diagnoses when confronted with a patient developing any type of rapidly progressive paralytic disease. Diplopia is one of the earliest manifestations of these diseases, and its association with any evidence of other muscle weakness should alert the physician to the possibility of the diagnosis and the potential need for respiratory care.

Drug Overdose

Drug overdose, particularly with narcotics, may lead to such rapid paralysis of the respiratory center that respiratory arrest is produced soon after loss of consciousness. Track marks on the arms and pinpoint pupils are clues to the diagnosis; if there is any doubt, a narcotic antagonist, naloxone for example, should be administered immediately. After administration of a narcotic antagonist, these patients may regain consciousness and even be able to answer questions, yet still have severe depression of respiration and a tendency to relapse into coma. They need to be watched closely until fully and permanently awake.

Asthma

It is uncommon for obstructive pulmonary disease to lead rapidly to respiratory arrest, but the one exception to this is asthma. There have been many instances in which patients with this condition were felt to have only mild airway obstruction, only to observe it progress to respiratory arrest in a matter of minutes. It is for this reason that all patients with asthma should be evaluated with measurements of expiratory flow rate; if the obstruction is severe, they must be promptly treated, often in an intensive respiratory care unit. It is remarkable how frequently patients are brought to the emergency room with respiratory arrest from asthma, intubated, and resuscitated, with prompt recovery and virtual disappearance of the signs of airway obstruction. Just as fatal bronchoconstriction with mucus plugging can develop with extraordinary rapidity, so may it disappear after loss of consciousness.

Pulmonary Edema

In other patients with asthma, or in patients with severe pulmonary edema with marked disturbance of lung mechanics, respiratory failure may result from respiratory muscle fatigue produced by the marked respiratory effort used to maintain ventilation. Prompt treatment of the underlying condition will usually prevent this progression, but it is a matter of delicate judgment as to when such patients should be intubated and given artificial ventilatory support. In severe *pulmonary edema*, froth and fluid may occlude most of the airways. Such patients may require intubation, suctioning, and artificial ventilation until the edema can be controlled.

UPPER AIRWAY OBSTRUCTION

Upper airway obstruction is a very special cause of respiratory arrest, and there are two particular situations in which recognition and treatment may be lifesaving.

Foreign Body

It is not uncommon for large morsels of food, particularly after the ingestion of alcohol, to become lodged in the upper airways. Typically an individual will be eating steak, rise from the table, and perhaps stagger from the room, only to fall to the ground or the floor apneic and unconscious. Dr. Henry Heimlich has called attention to this problem and pointed out that the appropriate treatment is to grasp the erect victim around the upper abdomen and apply a sudden compressive squeeze, thereby generating increased abdominal and thoracic pressure, which will forcefully expel the obstructing material from the mouth. A great many lives have been saved by the prompt application of the Heimlich maneuver in individuals who have aspirated steak, water, peanut butter, and a variety of other materials. Heimlich has pointed out that one should not attempt to dislodge the obstruction for fear that it will be forced further into the airway; rather, one should immediately apply this sudden jolt of compressive pressure so as to dislodge the object.

Epiglottitis

Epiglottitis is the other acute emergency that warrants special mention. Although it occurs most commonly in children, it also occurs in adults and is almost always associated with a very severe sore throat, usually accompanied by fever. Upper airway obstruction is generally associated with stridor, but this may proceed very rapidly, in a matter of minutes, to total obstruction. The inflammatory process may be so severe that intubation is extremely difficult, and if this is the case, immediate tracheostomy is mandatory. Thus, the physician should be alert to the fact that any difficulty in breathing or stridor in a patient with a severe sore throat warrants immediate attention and consideration of this potentially fatal but totally reversible disease.

Life-threatening upper airway obstruction may also develop from injury to the larynx, as from burns or from the laryngeal edema of acute anaphylaxis, such as from bee stings or administration of drugs to a sensitive subject.

DYSPNEA

Evaluation of the patient with dyspnea can present a great many problems. Obstructive airways disease, usually evident from physical examination and certainly from physiological study, may be a feature of pulmonary congestion ("cardiac asthma"), and the characteristic inspiratory crackles of pulmonary edema may be mimicked by diffuse interstitial disease of the lung. Careful examination, appropriate spirometric study, and, if necessary, evaluation of the response to therapy are important leads to the proper diagnosis.

Pulmonary Embolism

Patients presenting suddenly with severe dyspnea represent a special problem. A large pulmonary embolus may cause pronounced reflex hyperventilation manifest in severe dyspnea and, if there is sufficient obstruction of the pulmonary circulation, systemic hypotension and shock associated with venous congestion. In the absence of such extensive involvement of the pulmonary circulation, however, the diagnosis may be extremely difficult. Careful examination of the legs, perhaps with Doppler flow studies, may reveal a potential source. Pleuritic pain may be present, and a variety of radiographic findings, particularly an elevated diaphragm or small pleural effusion, may be evident, but the x-ray film of the chest may also be normal. Thus, severe dyspnea associated with hyperventilation may be the sole manifestation of a major pulmonary embolus, and suspicion of the diagnosis must lead to immediate perfusion scan and, possibly, angiography.

Spontaneous Pneumothorax

Another important cause of sudden dyspnea is a spontaneous pneumothorax. This may be associated with diminished breath sounds on the affected side, but not always. If there is sufficient accumulation of air to cause mediastinal swing, or tension pneumothorax, it should be possible to detect deviation of the trachea by placing the thumb in the suprasternal notch. However, the physical findings may not be obvious, and an x-ray film of the chest is obviously essential in any patient who presents with the sudden onset of shortness of breath. In the rare emergency of a tension pneumothorax causing respiratory and circulatory embarrassment, the physician may be forced to take immediate action by inserting a needle into an anterior intercostal space so as to remove the air, which will gush forth audibly under increased pressure. This may be followed by insertion of a plastic catheter into the pleural space in order to allow expansion of the lung without the danger of laceration. A pneumothorax can be evacuated by allowing the air to leave the chest during expiration, and then occluding the needle or plastic cannula as the lung expands during inspiration. The catheter can be connected to an underwater seal, so that if air does accumulate under pressure, it will bubble forth. Expansion will be aided by having the patient cough or make forceful expirations, generating a positive expiratory pressure, and the water seal will prevent any aspiration of air during the subsequent inspiration.

Hyperventilation Syndrome

Although not strictly a medical emergency, the hyperventilation syndrome may be confused with more severe illness. It is generally associated with symptoms of acute alkalosis, such as numbness and tingling in the extremities or lips. Respirations are apt to be irregular, with frequent sighs and yawns; and the patient often complains of an inability to take a deep breath rather than of a sustained shortness of breath. Measurement of blood gases reveals a low Pco_2 with respiratory alkalosis, no different from that associated with hyperventilation from many other causes, but the arterial oxygen tension is correspondingly elevated because the lungs are normal. In contrast to pulmonary edema or pulmonary embolism, there should be no increase of the alveolar-arterial oxygen gradient.

There are other interesting problems that may be associated with acute hyperventilation. If a person overbreathes, the Pco_2 is reduced, leading to dissociation of carbonic acid and excretion of bicarbonate stores from the blood and other organs. Because of the alkalosis, the normal stimulus to respiration is lost, and it will not be restored until the carbon dioxide stores are built up once again. As a result, after hyperventilation there is no feeling of a need to breathe and an individual can hold his breath for long periods of time. After prolonged, severe hyperventilation, for example, the breath may be held for several minutes before CO_2 stores once again build up to the point of a normal Pco_2, with restoration of the normal drive to breathe. This has two important practical consequences. Although CO_2 stores are built up slowly, oxygen is utilized during the period the breath is held. Since there is no corresponding pool of extra oxygen available in the body, rapidly progressive hypoxemia develops as soon as the oxygen in the lung is consumed. This may be associated with relatively little respiratory distress, and it is possible to hold the breath to the point of dangerous hypoxia with loss of consciousness. This is a matter of considerable concern in individuals who hyperventilate in an effort to perform a prolonged underwater swim, since they may lose consciousness before the need to breathe forces them to rise to the surface. The other practical consequence is that if patients are over-ventilated during resuscitation or by a respirator, the CO_2 stores are reduced; and when the artificial respiration is stopped, lack of spontaneous respiration may not reflect pulmonary derangement but may simply be a manifestation of the absence of the respiratory stimulus. Thus, after cessation of artificial respiration the patient should be observed for two or three minutes before concluding that spontaneous respiration will not resume.

ASPIRATION PNEUMONIA

The aspiration of gastric contents, as in elderly or obtunded patients, is a potentially devastating pulmonary insult. Such an event may lead to a rapidly progressive chemical pneumonitis, with adult respiratory distress and an extremely high mortality despite supportive care in a respiratory care unit. Another group of patients will develop a pneumonic lesion that slowly clears over several days. A third, important group appears to improve after the initial aspiration, only in a few days to develop progressive pneumonia, which is probably due to superimposed infection. There is also a high mortality in this group of patients, but it has been shown that prophylactic treatment with corticosteroids and antibiotics is without value.

The most important aspect of therapy of aspiration pneumonia is prevention. Patients who have difficulty swallowing must be carefully observed and fed slowly in small amounts. It is wise to have elderly patients sit erect for at least 1 to 2 hours after eating. The treatment of respiratory failure is supportive, and treatment of superimposed pneumonia depends upon identification of the infecting organism by examination of sputum or of material obtained by nasotracheal aspiration or even by lung puncture if necessary.

HEMOPTYSIS

Blood-streaked sputum is a very common symptom of bronchitis, pneumonia, tuberculosis, lung cancer, and many other pulmonary diseases. It must always be taken seriously and the correct diagnosis established by appropriate study. Massive hemoptysis, the expectoration of several hundred cubic centimeters of pure blood, is far less common and requires special consideration.

It is essential to make certain that the patient has actually coughed the blood from the lungs and that the bleeding is not from the upper airways or gastrointestinal tract. This may require otolaryngologic examination, and exclusion of bleeding from esophageal varices or peptic ulcer may be difficult unless the patient is actually observed to cough. One should remember that hemoptysis may be associated with swallowing of large amounts of blood, so that the gastric contents may have a coffee-ground appearance and be guaiac positive.

In patients with massive hemoptysis, there is almost always a visible lesion on the x-ray film of the chest. Only rarely is bronchitis associated with major bleeding. If bronchiectasis, which may cause severe hemorrhage from the increased bronchial collateral circulation, is the cause, there should be chronic changes evident on the roentgenogram. Most commonly, severe hemoptysis is due to cavitary disease of the lung, either a lung abscess, necrotizing carcinoma, or tuberculosis. The immediate priority in management is to establish control of the bleeding. This is done by positioning the patient in the most appropriate manner. There is no good information as to the best way to position the patient with a lung abscess; but it is probably wise, in the presence of active bleeding, to adopt a position in which the abscess is dependent, so that the cavity will become filled with blood and the bleeding will stop. The patient should be encouraged to cough gently in order to maintain patency of the airways, but a dry hacking cough may aggravate the bleeding and can be effectively suppressed by codeine. Even in the case of chronic tuberculous cavities, superimposed bacterial infection is usually the immediate cause of major bleeding, and broad-spectrum antibiotics should always be given to a patient with major hemoptysis.

In most cases, the bleeding will subside, and it will be possible to evaluate the cause and institute appropriate therapy, for tuberculosis, lung abscess, or bronchogenic carcinoma. If bleeding continues, one may have to consider emergency resection. Again, the guidelines are not clear, but the major indication for surgery is continued bleeding despite medical therapy. Bleeding may not always be evident as expectoration of blood but may be reflected in an increase in the size of an air fluid level in a cavity or in the appearance of new infiltrates in the lung, a sign of aspiration of blood and an indication that surgery may be necessary to order to prevent respiratory insufficiency. The combined judgment of the internist and thoracic surgeon is needed to evaluate this difficult problem. It is worth mentioning that in most cases of fatal hemoptysis, in which death is due to aspiration of blood with respiratory insufficiency rather than severe blood loss, the hemorrhage occurs so rapidly as to make any kind of treatment impossible. Once the bleeding has occurred, the major risk is past, and the physician must be concerned to institute the type of treatment least likely to be associated with future problems. Thus, if there is evidence of continued bleeding, it may be properly decided that an emergency lobectomy is associated with less risk than continued observation.

A major cause of severe hemorrhage is the aspergilloma, or fungus ball, which grows in the walls of a tuberculous or nontuberculous lung cavity. In patients with localized disease, this lesion is so apt to continue to bleed heavily, with a lethal outcome, that resection is probably indicated. But most of these lesions occur in patients with extensive pulmonary insufficiency due to underlying disease, and the risk of resection is prohibitive.

When surgery is not feasible, it may be possible to control the bleeding by insertion of a balloon catheter through a bronchoscope so as to tamponade the bleeding segment and allow the blood to clot, halting spread to other parts of the lung. Other approaches have included occlusion of the pulmonary artery supplying the bleeding segment or embolization of the bronchial arterial circulation to the infected lung. The former is often unsuccessful because the systemic bronchial circulation is the source of bleeding, and the latter approach may be complicated by embolization of a spinal artery, so that it must be done by skilled, experienced personnel.

After the risk of severe hemorrhage has subsided, it is important to establish the cause of bleeding. In some cases, underlying disease, such as mitral stenosis, pneumonia, pulmonary infarction or the alveolar hemorrhage associated with Goodpasture's syndrome, other collagen vascular disease, or lung trauma, may be quite evident. In other cases, bronchoscopy is indicated and should be timed so as to reveal the site of the bleeding even if a specific diagnosis cannot be made. Thus, bronchoscopy is generally performed as the bleeding is subsiding but before it has stopped completely, so that it will be possible to visualize the blood coming from a specific segment of the lung. This is particularly important in view of the possible need for emergency surgery at a later date.

The major causes of hemoptysis are listed in Table 10–1. The diagnosis can generally be made by appropriate radiographic and bronchoscopic study. Often bronchography is necessary to reveal a small area of bronchiectasis associated with pulmonary hemorrhage. In many other cases the diagnosis of bronchitis-bronchiectasis is made if the patient is a smoker and

Table 10–1   Causes of Hemoptysis

Bronchitis–bronchiectasis
Bronchogenic carcinoma (adenoma)
Tuberculosis (usually cavitary)
Lung abscess
Infected cyst (asporgilloma)
Pulmonary venous hypertension (mitral stenosis)
Pulmonary AV fistula
Alveolar hemorrhage (Goodpasture's syndrome)
Pneumonia
Calcified hilar lymph node
Pulmonary infarction

no other lesion is found after careful study. Most of these conditions have been considered previously, but it is worth noting that a calcified hilar lymph node, often a result of old tuberculosis or histoplasmosis, can erode into a bronchus and cause severe hemoptysis. There have been reports of recurrent hemoptysis at the time of menstruation, possibly related to endometriosis, and it has been said that bronchial adenomas, so prevalent in young women, are particularly likely to bleed at this time.

PLEURAL EFFUSION

Pleural effusion is rarely a medical emergency, though it may signify serious disease urgently requiring diagnosis and appropriate therapy. One exception is the pleural effusion or hydropneumothorax that may result from *rupture of the esophagus*. This is a potentially lethal illness and often follows forceful vomiting, though it may be the result of trauma and can even occur at rest. It most commonly follows esophagoscopy. Patients are usually acutely ill, with high fever. They may have subcutaneous emphysema, but often not until several hours after the rupture. The pleural effusion is usually on the left, but it may be on the right, is rarely bilateral, and may not become evident until the mediastinitis extends into the pleural space. Pleural fluid with a pH less then 6.0 or with a very high concentration of amylase, which is of salivary origin, is practically diagnostic. Barium contrast study should be performed to make a precise diagnosis, and immediate thoracotomy is mandatory. Untreated, the mortality is extremely high, but surgical drainage is usually succesful.

SUPERIOR VENA CAVA SYNDROME

The sudden appearance of facial swelling and edema is strongly suggestive of occlusion of the superior vena cava, most commonly from bronchogenic carcinoma but also from lymphoma or mediastinitis. This is frequently very frightening to patient and to physician, but is usually not of life-threatening severity, even though it may be associated with increased intracranial pressure. The diagnosis should be made promptly, if necessary by venography and mediastinotomy, so as to institute radiotherapy, perhaps in combination with chemotherapy, if a tumor is present.

SMOKE INHALATION

Victims of smoke inhalation may suffer from a number of problems. Immediately after exposure, particularly if it is associated with intense heat and facial burns, they may develop acute laryngeal edema requiring intubation or a tracheostomy. Four to 24 hours later injury to the lung may be evident as pulmonary edema, and careful observation is needed for 24 hours to detect and treat this form of the adult respiratory distress syndrome. After a latent period of up to seven days, injury to the airways may become evident as the necrotic epithelium and excessive secretions accumulate and move up the mucociliary escalator. This is usually a self-limited problem, although it may be associated with wheeze and dyspnea. At any time after the damage to lung or airways, superinfection may develop, and this must be promptly identified and treated with the appropriate antibiotics. However, as in other case of diffuse lung injury, there is no indication for the use of prophylactic antibiotics or corticosteroids.

Carbon Monoxide Poisoning

Carbon monoxide (CO) poisoning is a special problem that results from the inhalation of fumes generated by the incomplete combustion of hydrocarbons, particularly gasoline. It is an insidious, painless, and lethal form of hypoxia. Carbon monoxide has an avid affinity for hemoglobin, preventing oxygen uptake by the blood and transport to the tissues. Victims of CO intoxication must be recognized and given oxygen just as soon as possible so that the increased alveolar Po_2 can successfully compete with the carbon monoxide for attachment to the hemoglobin molecule. In the meantime, artificial ventilation must be instituted so as to wash the carbon monoxide out of the lungs.

All smokers suffer from some degree of chronic carbon monoxide poisoning, and this may be one of the reasons why they are particularly vulnerable to the myocardial ischemia caused by coronary artery occlusion. Carbon monoxide levels are unacceptably high in many urban areas, particularly during periods of atmospheric inversion when stagnant air results in accumulation of automobile emissions in the atmosphere. The effects are chronic rather than acute and rarely dangerous.

DROWNING

Death from drowning is the result of asphyxia either from displacement of air in the lungs by water or from reflex laryngospasm secondary to aspiration of water. The immediate priority of management is use of the Heimlich maneuver to expel water from the lungs and initiation of mouth-to-mouth resuscitation to provide effective alveolar ventilation. Drowning victims should be transported to an intensive care unit for artificial ventilation through an endotracheal tube for as long as is necessary and maintained there for careful observation for the development of complications. Fresh-water drowning may be associated with marked hyponatremia and hemolysis because of the absorption of hypotonic fluid into the circulation, whereas salt-water drowning is characterized by hypernatremia. These disturbances are generally self-limited and do not require special therapy. The lung is, however, vulnerable to secondary infection, and careful observation for the development of fever, new infiltrates, or purulent sputum is important. Prophylactic antibiotics should not be used, but infections should be promptly treated after the causative organism has been identified. There is no evidence that corticosteroids are of value.

Additional Reading

Bynum LJ, Pierce HK: Pulmonary aspiration of gastric contents. Am Rev Resp Dis 114:1129–1136, 1975.

Goff AM, Gaensler EA: Hyperventilation syndrome. Respiration 26:359, 1969.

Heimlich HJ: The Heimlich maneuver: where it stands today. Emergency Med 10:89, 1978.

Modell JH, Graves SA, Ketover A: Clinical course of 91 consecutive near-drowning victims. Chest 70:231–239, 1976.

Saw EC, Gottlieb LS, Yokayama T, et al: Flexible fiberoptic bronchoscopy and endobronchial tamponade in the management of massive hemoptysis. Chest 70:589–591, 1976.

INDEX

Page numbers in *italics* refer to illustrations. Page numbers followed by (t) refer to tables.